PRAISE FOR *SKINCARE FOR YOUR SOUL*

"To those of us who fell (happily) into the Asian skincare rabbit hole, Jude is better known as Fiddy Snails. If not for her research, breaking down what seemed like an extremely complex skincare routine to skincare newbies all around the world, most of us would have never discovered the joy from a skincare routine. If not for her, neither would many K-beauty brands be known across the world. Jude has generously shared all her time and years' worth of knowledge—her work rings of honesty and integrity. You need this book."

—**Chinmayi Sripaada**, singer, voice actor, and entrepreneur

"A truly beautiful and informative book about self-care as much as it is about skincare. An absolute holy grail for your library, *Skincare for Your Soul* makes skincare accessible for everyone from curious newbies to the most ardent enthusiasts. Jude generously shares her knowledge to help you make your skincare work better for you."

—**Ann Shen**, bestselling author of *Nevertheless, She Wore It*

"Give a woman a moisturizer and she will glow for a day; teach a woman to select a moisturizer based on active ingredients, her skin type, and mental health needs, and she will glow for the rest of her life! Whether you are a skincare newbie or a longtime veteran (who survived the age of St. Ives Apricot Scrub), Jude Chao's prose is like chatting with a caring best friend who just happens to understand what 'stratum corneum' means. Between the illuminating scientific deep dives, Jude generously shares her personal story of how washing her face for thirty seconds a day evolved into using skin care as a powerful tool for improving her mental health. *Skin Care for Your Soul* cuts through all the BS of marketing and ridiculous beauty standards of this FaceTuned era and guides you through creating a routine that will benefit YOU specifically, in your mind and body. Bonus: your moisture barrier will be pretty pleased, too."

—**Christina Wolfgram**, comedian, mental health enthusiast, and host of *Sobcast the Podcast*

"This book feels like talking with a trusted friend, one so generous with practical advice and wisdom. I wish our Dermatology textbooks had chapters like these!"

—**Dr. Erin Tababa-Santos**, creator of The Nerdy Derma

Skin Care

FOR YOUR SOUL

Skin Care

FOR YOUR SOUL

Achieving *Outer Beauty* and
Inner Peace with Korean Skincare

Jude Chao

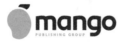
mango
PUBLISHING GROUP

CORAL GABLES

Cover and Interior Layout Design: Jermaine Lau

Published by Mango Publishing, a division of Mango Media Inc.

Mango is an active supporter of authors' rights to free speech and artistic expression in their books. The purpose of copyright is to encourage authors to produce exceptional works that enrich our culture and our open society. Uploading or distributing photos, scans or any content from this book without prior permission is theft of the author's intellectual property.
Please honor the author's work as you would your own. Thank you in advance for respecting our authors' rights.

For permission requests, please contact the publisher at:

Mango Publishing Group
2850 Douglas Road, 2nd Floor
Coral Gables, FL 33134 USA
info@mango.bz

For special orders, quantity sales, course adoptions and corporate sales, please email the publisher at sales@mango.bz. For trade and wholesale sales, please contact Ingram Publisher Services at customer.service@ingramcontent.com or +1.800.509.4887.

Skincare for Your Soul: Achieving Outer Beauty and Inner Peace with Korean Skincare

ISBN: (p) 978-1-64250-494-1

BIASC: HEA003000—HEALTH & FITNESS / Beauty & Grooming

LCCN: Pending

This book is not intended as a substitute for the medical advice of physicians. The reader should regularly consult a physician/dermatologist in matters relating to his/her health and skin and particularly with respect to any symptoms that may require diagnosis or medical attention. The author and publisher advise readers to take full responsibility for their safety.

Printed in the United States of America.

For my family,

without whom neither I nor this book would be here.
All of you have shaped me and made me who I am,
and I hope I make you proud.

TABLE OF CONTENTS

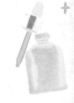

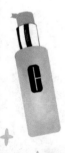

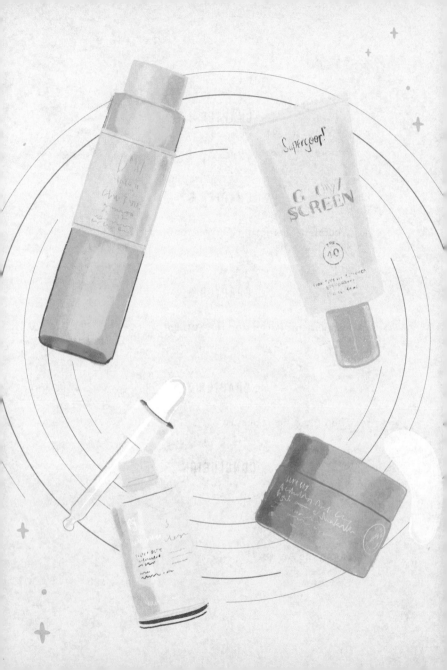

FOREWORD

The first time I came across Jude's glorious blog *Fifty Shades of Snail*, I knew we were kindred skincare spirits. Our virtual meet happened as I was on a quest to find information on an obscure Taiwanese essence, and the only review that came up at the time was Jude's. And you know what they say about great minds. I quickly became consumed by her reviews, engaged by her personality and knowledge, and discovered, as it turns out, we wholly share the same point of view, which is a rare, rare thing in my life. I may have even burst into open applause while reading... alone in silence.

I'm probably most captivated by her snarky sensibility and provoking quirkiness which catches like wildfire across the skincare community. She's reframed pores into "face sphincters," advocates a practical "three finger" sunscreen application method, claims rubber masks are exactly 35 percent scarier than clay ones, and calls out inappropriately-translated, racist-sounding product names. Even though Jude has done time in the beauty industry herself, and is therefore able to discern the difference between a marketing headline, superficial trends, and the real deal formulas, she never pontificates or comes off as didactic or preachy. So yes, she's smart as hell, but sounds more like a friend than a know-it-all.

After actually getting to know Jude, however, I was still struck by how well her perspective resonates with my own—our conversations are wide-ranging, from food porn to life-views to the purpose of things. Not only did I discover a fellow treasure hunter in the all-too-often overhyped and oversaturated world of beauty, I also learned that she experienced a powerful journey in becoming who she is today. It is one that she shares beautifully and honestly in this book.

Reviewing skincare is also what I do as *Gothamista* on YouTube. My approach is not about telling people what to do—judging or scolding the skincare choices of others—and it's most definitely not about devising extensive skincare to-do lists. If you want those things, I have a fabulous and very bossy Eastern European esthetician who will berate you while giving you the most glorious facial. Skincare for me is intuitive, an expression of self-love, and thus it is inherently therapeutic. I get excited about new formulas and look forward to my daily ritual. And this is precisely where Jude and I fully align. There are few voices that I trust and listen to as intently to be steered in the right direction. In fact, I am far too easily enabled by anything bearing Jude's seal of approval.

Skincare for the Soul speaks to me. It is a journey into skincare discovery, but it is also a voyage into the mind and our sense of self. Jude is your honest and upfront friend with simple, intuitive guidance without judgment. This book is not just a guide full of treasured nuggets of good sense, but at its "essence" (see what I did there?), it's an accessible and encouraging resource for those just wading into skincare and looking for direction and truth, as well as for those who are already deeper in. You may just find your skincare soulmate here, too. Enjoy!

RENÉE

Gothamista

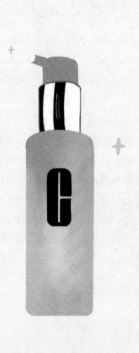

MORE THAN SKIN DEEP

It started with a bar of Clinique facial soap in a pale green plastic case and a bottle of fragrant pink Oil of Olay "Beauty Fluid." Those products—my adoptive mom's skincare staples back in the 1980s—lodged themselves in my consciousness as my first clear beauty memories. They sent me down a path I didn't even know I was walking until nearly thirty years later.

As a kid, I admired and aspired to my mom's meticulous beauty routine. As one of only a few Asians in our midsized Midwestern town, she already stood out, but she stood out even more because of the care she took with her appearance—not to fit in, but to look her best, always. She kept it up as much as she could even when cancer put her in the hospital; she kept it up as much as she could even when chemotherapy claimed her hair. Wigs gave her back her chic Sheena Easton haircut. Ill for many years of my childhood, she cleansed and moisturized, selected her earrings with care, swiped on vibrant lipsticks, and collected department store gift-with-purchase makeup bags and eyeshadow palettes from her favorite beauty brands.

I didn't get it then. I was too young. I took her rituals for granted: I thought that that's just how she was, that it didn't go deeper than that.

She died when I was thirteen, but her habits stuck with me. I always wanted to take care of my skin the way she'd taken care of hers, to treat myself as well as she did, because that's how she was and how I wanted to be. At the time, I didn't assign skincare any more meaning than that, but that was enough to keep me invested. As a teenager, I fumbled through Noxzema cleansing creams, harsh Buf Puf exfoliators, and tube after tube of the notoriously abrasive St. Ives apricot scrub. A broke student in my twenties, I washed my face with whatever cleanser was on sale when I needed one, occasionally exfoliated with scrubby shower gloves, and splurged on Olay moisturizers with SPF.

It wasn't until I hit my thirties, chronically overexfoliated and sporting patches of melasma from too much sun and too little SPF while pregnant, that I finally understood what this ritual meant to me. Not just what kinds of products to use or in what order and quantity, but why.

My mom's beauty regimen was not just about looking prettier. Results are great, and results are something to strive for, but it's the act of skincare itself that matters. And though she has been gone for a very long time and I can't ask her to confirm, I think she would agree. Surely she knew no one would judge her appearance when she was sick. But keeping up the routine was an expression of optimism and an act of care for herself—a way of asserting who she was, even when illness threatened to take that away.

I have been lucky in my physical health so far—luckier than my mom was at my age—but I know the fear of losing my *self*, in my case to depression.

I was diagnosed at twenty years old with major depressive disorder, but looking back at my teenage years, I believe I had been suffering from it for several years by then. And despite my diagnosis, I would continue to suffer from it for the next decade or so. My experience with depression, and realization of how much my skincare routine helped me stay centered, inspired me to write an essay for the website Fashionista. In it, I wrote:

Depression isn't about feeling sad all the time, at least not for me. That would require giving a shit. My depression manifests as being unable to give a shit. In fact, when I'm in the depths of a depressive episode, I can't even give a shit about not giving a shit, no matter how much I know I really should give a shit. The days blur together until I wake up one day and realize that I've lost another six months or another year, my life and sense of self stolen right out from under my nose, again.

Day to day, I functioned well enough to maintain relationships (more or less) and to keep jobs (more or less), but for much of my adult life, I existed in a fog, sometimes medicated, sometimes unmedicated, sometimes self-medicated, always detached from myself. I enjoyed very little, felt in control of nothing, and made bad choices.

Skincare changed that for me and for many people I've spoken to over the years. I'm here to tell you why and show you how.

Before we start, though, please remember that I am not a doctor. I'm a layperson whose interest in skincare led me down a rabbit hole of research. I've spent countless hours reading other laypeople's experiences and anecdotes, puzzling over peer-reviewed studies on skin function and responses to cosmetic ingredients, and chatting with fellow skincare enthusiasts as well as professional cosmetic chemists and dermatologists. All that research has informed my blog, *Fifty Shades of Snail*, which I've written since 2015, and it informs my product reviews and recommendations, but at the end of the day, I am not a doctor. Nor am I here to police your choices for your skin— only to give you ideas of where to start and how to figure out where to go.

I'm not a therapist either, and I am not recommending skincare as a substitute for professional psychiatric care and medication as needed. I am also not recommending the act of purchasing skincare as a sort of retail therapy. There will be no product recommendations in this book. In fact, we'll discuss manipulative and exploitative skincare marketing tactics to look out for.

I'm a person who has suffered from depression and anxiety for my entire adult life, and who has found greater peace and resilience (and better skin!) through skincare. What I've learned and shared along the way has resonated with many of the people who've joined me on this journey, and I'm here to share it with you, too.

I recommend skincare as an extra tool in your arsenal against depressive episodes, downward spirals of anxiety, and whatever else you may be facing. I'm writing this in 2020, when many of us are facing challenges we've never experienced before. The global pandemic and ensuing economic chaos have exacerbated many people's existing struggles while giving others their first experience of true existential dread. So much of our lives is out of our control, and so many of us need to find some way to take back control in whatever ways we can.

If you're looking for ways to take better care of yourself from the inside out, I can show you how to elevate your everyday beauty routine into an affirmation of your value. When everything feels like a drag and nothing seems worth the effort, skincare can be a lifeline to cling to as you make your way back to shore.

If you're just looking for ways to improve your skin's appearance without resorting to lasers, knives, injectables, and other invasive and expensive treatments, I can show you how to do that, too. Contrary to what some in the industry claim, you can achieve dramatic results without going under the knife or needle. It takes more time, more patience, and the right products for your skin, but it is absolutely doable. I would even argue that achieving improvements without medical interventions is healthier for the soul, thanks to the satisfaction of knowing that you did it all yourself.

Your skincare routine can be a daily act of care for yourself that will yield visible improvements to your appearance while calming and grounding your mind. A journey of discovery and, for some of you, a key to a warm and welcoming community like no other. I'm here to give you the tools to get you started on your way.

Skincare isn't magic. Nothing is. But it has changed my life and the lives of others in ways that go far beyond how our faces look.

Sometimes, it really is that deep.

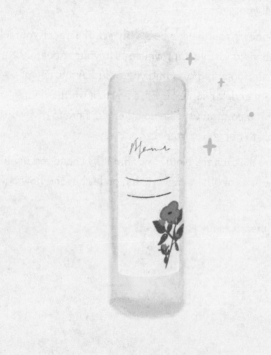

Chapter 1

GETTING STARTED

When setting out on any journey, it's best to know where you're starting from and where you plan to end up—this will help you avoid too many unnecessary detours and delays on your path. Having a clear idea of your needs and goals will also help minimize your expenses. Your skincare options these days are nearly endless; narrowing your choices down as much as possible from the start will minimize your chances of buying products that aren't suitable for you.

To start off on the right foot, you should first identify your skin type, then any skin conditions you may have. Use your skin type to determine which types of products will likely benefit you the most. Use your skin condition to learn which types of ingredients you should seek out or avoid.

YOUR SKIN TYPE

Thanks to mainstream beauty marketing, you're most likely already aware of the concept of skin types. We inherit our skin type, which indicates our skin's natural oil production tendencies and reactiveness to external stimuli.

While age, hormones, and some medications can alter our skin type, most topically applied, non-prescription cosmetic ingredients won't. Consistent use of products appropriate for our needs can compensate for deficiencies and minimize imbalances to optimize the function and outward appearance of our skin, however.

Knowing your skin type will give you a better understanding of why your skin behaves the way it does and provide a general guide to the types of products and ingredients that stand the best chance of benefiting you. You don't need to adhere rigidly to skin type distinctions, though. There's a tendency towards dogmatic thinking in skincare communities and marketing, the idea that certain products should only be used by the skin types indicated on their labels. "Best for [X skin type]" language is easy shorthand to help consumers make purchasing decisions but shouldn't be taken as absolute law.

Some of my favorite products overlap with those of friends who have drastically different skin types than I do. The differences lie more in *how* we use those products. I have normal skin that can get dry, depending on the weather or how much I've overused a tantalizing exfoliant in recent days. Stacking multiple products works well for me. Someone with oilier skin may not layer as many in a single routine as I do. There are products that benefit us both; we just use them in different ways.

You don't need to only use the products and ingredients marketed as suitable for your skin type. Consider them a starting point and work from there.

Dry

Dry skin doesn't produce enough oil to keep its upper layers lubricated and protected against moisture loss from within. If your skin has pretty much always felt tight and uncomfortable, this may be you. Another tell of dry skin is small to invisible pore size.

Normal

Normal skin is, well, normal. Moisture levels maintain a more or less optimal balance. Skin doesn't feel tight or dry, nor does it feel oily.

Oily

Oily skin, as you might guess, overproduces oil. This is pretty unmistakable. Your skin tends to get oily quickly, and pore size is often enlarged.

Combination

Combination skin has zones of different skin types: maybe an oily T-zone and dry cheeks, or normal cheeks and dry T-zone, or any other permutation. Each zone will follow the general preferences of its skin type.

Sensitive

Any of the above skin types can also be sensitive. Sensitive skin reacts more often and usually more intensely to irritants and/or physical touch. Some common triggers are fragrance, alcohol, exfoliants, certain detergents, certain preservatives, and certain botanical extracts and oils. If your skin is predisposed to sensitivity, you've most likely experienced reactions since childhood. Reactions can take the form of redness, flushing, pain and stinging, or even welts and rashes.

Acne-Prone

Any of the above skin types can also be more predisposed to breakouts. These might be caused by certain cosmetic ingredients; by lifestyle factors like dirty pillowcases, poor air quality, or diet; or by hormones. Hormonal acne or acne caused or worsened by your diet calls for a visit to a doctor.

Once you've identified your skin type, make a note of it. But skin type is just the beginning. Once you know your skin type, you can refine your choices further by considering your current skin condition, which we'll discuss below.

YOUR SKIN CONDITION

In contrast to skin type, which is inherited and largely fixed, your skin condition is caused by external factors. Skin conditions can cause some confusion, because their symptoms often mimic skin types, but unlike skin type, skin conditions can be changed.

Dehydrated

In my conversations with my blog readers and social media followers over the years, the topic of dehydrated skin has come up again and again. Characterized by accelerated water loss through the uppermost layers of skin, dehydrated skin occurs when skin's moisture barrier—which protects against moisture loss and external irritants and contaminants—is compromised, something we'll discuss in detail in the chapters about cleansing and about exfoliation.

One of the most common tells of dehydrated skin is excessive oiliness at the surface, paired with a tight, dry sensation underneath. Lipids are leaking out of the normal structure of the moisture barrier, creating an oil slick on top of the skin but failing to hold in the moisture within. Not all dehydrated skin presents as oily on the outside and parched on the inside, though. Dehydrated skin can also appear the same as inherently dry skin.

If you suspect that you have dehydrated skin, take a close look at its texture. Dehydrated skin tends to look crepey due to a lack of water to plump it up at the surface. If you gently press your fingertip into your cheek, you'll likely see fine lines radiating outwards from where you're applying pressure. Dehydrated skin also lacks the ability to bounce back quickly from a poke or a pinch.

Sensitized

The signs of sensitized skin mimic those of genetically sensitive skin: unpleasant reactions to certain ingredients, products, or even touch. Sensitized skin generally reacts to the same kinds of triggers as genetically sensitive skin, too. Where sensitized and sensitive skin differ is in their origin. Sensitive skin has always been that way. Sensitized skin, on the other hand, develops due to an outside influence, like exposure to a particular sensitizing agent, or weakening of the moisture barrier.

Congested

Most of us have experienced the occasional breakout.
Something has clogged our pores or caused infection.
Sometimes skin grows over the clog, forming the closed,
colorless bumps called closed comedones. Other times, the
clog becomes inflamed, leading to the classic red, swollen
pimple. Congestion happens even to people whose skin
isn't acne-prone. Usually it comes from using some product
or ingredient that doesn't agree with our skin, but it can
also occur due to a weakened moisture barrier.

* * *

As you might have noticed, all three of these common skin
conditions are often rooted in a damaged moisture barrier.
In chapter three, we'll talk about your cleansing routine,
which can have a profound effect on the health of your
barrier. For now, it's enough to have a general idea of what
your skin type and condition may be. You'll be creating
your routine gradually, one step and product at a time.
Along the way, you'll learn more about your skin and what
works for it (and doesn't) on an individual level. Skincare
isn't one size fits all.

ON BEAUTY STANDARDS AND SETTING REALISTIC GOALS

After reading the last section, you've probably spent some time thinking about the appearance of your skin and maybe looking more closely at it in the mirror. That's why we're going to take a minute now to talk about beauty standards and the power that a realistic (or unrealistic) goal can have over us.

Now more than ever, we are bombarded on all sides by images of absolutely flawless skin. Those of us old enough to remember getting all our beauty advice from glossy magazines will also remember how frustrated we felt when nothing we ever did actually produced the perfect skin we saw in the pages of *Seventeen, YM, Vogue, Elle, W*, and *Bazaar*. Older now, we know that those images were professionally retouched and not a representation of reality.

Yeah, well. The days of feeling bad about our skin because we were comparing ourselves to the flawlessly porcelain complexions of 1990s supermodels like Shalom Harlow seem like quaint olden times now, in the era of Instagram, FaceTune, Meitu, Snow, and other photo editing apps.

Back in the old days, we knew advertising was deceptive. Corporations presented unattainable images of beauty in order to make consumers feel insecure and thus sell them more products to assuage that insecurity. That's capitalism, and after a certain point, we can at least recognize it, even if we may not succeed in tuning its influence out completely.

These days, however, it can feel like *everyone* is presenting an impossibly flawless appearance to the world. It's not just the model Linda Evangelista on a magazine cover. Non-celebrities living perfectly ordinary lives post selfies featuring skin as smooth as heavy cream. Not a blemish dots the face of that one girl you knew in high school and still follow on social media fifteen years later. Your first boyfriend's mom appears to have aged backwards in the decades since you last saw her.

Yes, some of the people abusing the beauty filters are doing so to sell a product or to monetize the concept of themselves as a product, but others don't seem to be selling anything by presenting an idealized version of themselves. And the fact that it *is* an idealized version may not be immediately obvious to a casual onlooker. Sometimes it just looks like everyone else has perfect everything.

Which is *completely* untrue.

The accessibility and ease of use of modern photo editing apps allows amateurs with no training in image retouching to achieve the kind of photographic perfection once only associated with celebrities and corporate advertising. Honestly, some people turn themselves into a completely different person in their photos. And while body retouching can be pretty obvious—most people don't have nineteen-inch waists paired with forty-five-inch hips, or legs that take up three quarters of their entire body length—skin retouching can be more insidious, because it *seems* plausible that someone could have completely poreless and smooth skin with no irregularities of texture or tone.

In order to make our skincare journey something that benefits our mental health and improves our lives, we have to let go of the idea that the end goal is filter-level skin. It is not.

In the vast, vast, vast majority of cases, that absolutely poreless, flawless, smooth, and even-toned skin is a lie.

It's the result of makeup, lighting, filters, and retouching. Judging our skin's progress and appearance based on how it compares to the beauty filter skin we see online will only bring discouragement and unhappiness.

The goal is not absolute perfection. The goal is to get our skin to the best condition it can be in, based on our individual circumstances and genetics, and to feel better about ourselves as we do so. As you find the products and practices that work best for you, your skin *will* improve. It may never become utterly Cover Girl flawless, but it will function and feel and look better than it does now. Then the goal is to maintain it in that state as much as reasonably possible.

"Reasonably" is the key word here.

Many of us who are drawn to skincare's potential as a self-care and mental health tool tend to be prone to anxious thought patterns and unhealthy self-talk. If undertaken without mindfulness, skincare can feed into this and become another source of anxiety, rather than a tool for managing it. This is something I've discussed fairly extensively on social media. I want to take some time to talk here about ways to recognize when your interest in skincare is turning into an unhealthy compulsion.

Unfortunately, there are a lot of echo chambers and influences online that can encourage compulsive or neurotic thinking around skincare.

If you start experiencing any of the following thoughts or patterns, reflect on whether you've started using skincare as an outlet for unhealthy compulsions:

- **Nitpicking the appearance of your skin:** It's good to be observant and recognize changes in your skin, whether positive or negative. It is not so good to be glued to your magnifying mirror, fretting over every bump, pore, and tiny irregularity you see. My usual advice is, if you don't need a magnifying mirror for vision impairment reasons, don't own them. No one has magnifying eyes. If you need a magnifying mirror to see that "blemish," then it isn't a blemish.

- **Thinking harshly about your skin:** "My skin looks terrible." "My acne is never going to go away." "I look gross." No. If you wouldn't say it to your friend and you wouldn't say it to your child, don't say it to yourself. Changing negative self-talk patterns is an important part of improving mental health, and it applies to our self-talk about skin, too. (And if you would say it to your friend or child, skincare is not your biggest problem.)

Extrapolating catastrophic effects from a failure to improve your skin: "No one is ever going to love me if my skin doesn't clear up"; "my partner is going to leave me for someone younger if he notices I'm starting to get fine lines." (Frankly, if your partner did, that would mean your partner was trash in the first place.) Ultimately, skin is skin. It will not determine the amount of love you receive, or the quality of your life, unless you allow it to by letting insecurities dictate your responses to others.

Becoming obsessive about certain aspects of your routine: This happens a lot with sunscreen. We know sunscreen is important for both health and beauty reasons, and we know proper care should be taken to apply it correctly and use it consistently. From there, it's unfortunately all too easy to go overboard and begin obsessing about it. I find myself fielding a lot of questions about the potentially deleterious effects of not always using enough sunscreen, or skipping skincare a few nights a week. There's even a micro-trend involving using sunscreen at night to protect against the blue light emitted by electronics screens. (For the record, I am not even a little bit concerned about the effect of my screens on my skin.)

If you find yourself having thoughts like these, remember that none of this is life or death. It's skincare. We're here because we want to improve our skin in a way that also enhances our mental health. We're not here to let our beauty routines turn into compulsions that take over our lives.

It all goes back to the expectations we set for ourselves. That's why I like to ask people to articulate exactly what they want to improve about their skin before I offer any advice. As you consider your goals, be as granular and specific as you can.

If you set your goal as "perfect skin," you'll never reach that goal—it doesn't exist. Every single person in the world can find at least one thing about their skin that they'd consider an imperfection. On top of that, skin is a part of our living body. It's always changing: shedding dead cells, generating new ones, altering over time.

The most exploitative and manipulative marketing tricks used by the beauty industry all hinge on the delusion of perfection: both its attainability (through the products being marketed) and its power (to bestow a more perfect life and perfect happiness on the possessor of "perfect" skin). Finding happiness in your skin demands a rejection of the pursuit of perfection.

Think in more specific terms, and don't set too many goals all at once. It is not realistic or helpful to decide you want "perfect skin." It *is* realistic and can be helpful to decide you'd like to:

- Minimize the appearance of enlarged pores
- Reduce the frequency and severity of breakouts
- Fade dark spots and hyperpigmentation
- Improve skin's firmness and texture
- Soften fine lines
- Protect skin from UV damage and delay the visible signs of skin aging

Goals like these are attainable. Now we can begin to discuss how.

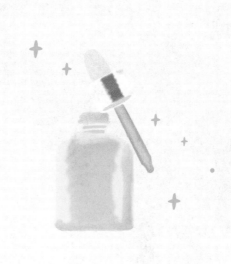

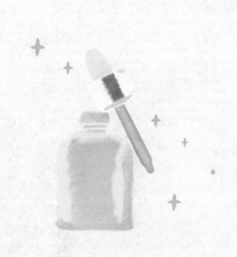

Chapter 2

WHAT TO KNOW BEFORE BUILDING A SKINCARE ROUTINE

Skincare these days is no simple thing. In the first decade of the 2000s, most of us in the Western world understood a skincare routine to consist of a cleanser, perhaps an astringent toner, and a moisturizer. It was hard to mix up the order in which to use those products. Some people might have added makeup remover and/or eye cream. The most complicated calculation most of us had to make was figuring out whether we really needed a separate day and night moisturizer. As for brands, they generally fell into three categories: bland but inoffensive dermatologist-recommended lines, basic drugstore lines, and higher-end department store and esthetician lines.

It's a whole different universe today. There are oil cleansers, foaming cleansers, gel cleansers, and micellar waters. The alcohol-laden astringent toners still exist, according to my last trip down a drugstore skincare aisle, but Asian beauty has brought hydrating toners into Western consciousness, and those are completely different from the Sea Breeze astringent we're used to. AHAs, BHAs, retinoids, and vitamin C serums (all of which we'll cover in a later chapter) promise to resurface and renew skin from the outside in and the inside out. There are essences, serums, ampoules, emulsions, and seemingly endless moisturizer options to seal them in. And that's before you even get into the nearly infinite array of masks. My evening routine rivals many spa facials, and I can do it every night if I want to.

No wonder many newcomers to skincare become quickly overwhelmed. Everything sounds important. Where are they supposed to start? Buy a prefab skincare routine? (Don't do that.) Copy their favorite skincare guru's routine? (Don't do that.) Personally choose a product in each category, buy them all at once, and start them all at once? (*Please* don't do that.)

Patience is key to curating a skincare routine that works best for you without subjecting your skin to multiple mysterious mishaps along the way. It's best to take it one product at a time.

To help you figure out in what order to assemble your routine, I've created a system similar to Maslow's Hierarchy of Needs, which organizes human needs and motivations into a five-tiered pyramid.

At the very base of the pyramid of Maslow's Hierarchy of Needs are physiological needs, encompassing basic survival necessities like food and water. Above physiological needs are safety needs like physical and emotional security. Next comes the need for social belonging: friendship, intimate relationships, and family. Higher still is self-esteem, which concerns itself with recognition, status, and respect. And at the top of the pyramid is self-actualization—the manifestation of one's true potential.

Within the skincare community, many people struggle with how to prioritize the different products in a skincare routine. Which should they tackle first—treatment products or basic care? If they don't have the budget for a comprehensive skincare routine, what should they focus on?

After thinking about and researching these questions for years, this is the skincare hierarchy of needs I've come up with.

SKINCARE HIERARCHY OF NEEDS

Refinement

Treatment

Protection

Sustenance

A HIERARCHY OF SKINCARE NEEDS

This hierarchy of skincare needs serves several purposes. It provides a framework for building your skincare routine in a way that helps to promote your overall skin health from the very beginning. It will also help you prioritize your skincare purchases.

1. Bottom Level: Sustenance

At the very base of the pyramid of my hierarchy of skincare needs, you'll find sustenance. These are the products that your skin needs in order to continue functioning correctly at a baseline level of health. Cleansers and moisturizers belong to this level.

2. Second Level: Protection

Above sustenance comes protection. Products that belong to this level actively defend skin from external factors that cause harm. On this level, you'll find sunscreen. Its protection will delay skin's deterioration due to age and extrinsic factors.

3. Third Level: Treatment

Above protection comes treatment. This level contains the ingredients shown to actively target and reduce or eliminate specific skin problems, such as visible skin aging, hyperpigmentation, acne, or excessive sensitivity and inflammation. Effective treatment products often change the very function and structure of skin—for example, retinoids accelerate and normalize skin regeneration, while niacinamide helps break up and disperse pigmentation deposits in skin.

4. Fourth and Top Level: Refinement

At the very top level of the pyramid is refinement. This level is for the perfectionists among us (or those for whom appearance is a job requirement). Products in the refinement category affect the appearance and sometimes the function of the very upper, most visible layers of skin. The best of the bunch can firm those upper layers of skin, creating a denser and more youthful appearance, or bring a radiant glow.

* * *

This hierarchy of needs can help clarify how you should prioritize your skincare choices. If you spend your time and money on refinement products without taking care of sustenance, protection, and treatment in order, you'll end up wasting a lot of money. The comparatively superficial and minor effects of even the best treatment products can't compensate for poor sustenance and protection. Meanwhile, if you focus on sustenance, protection, and treatment, your skin will look and feel much better than before, even if you don't spend time or money on refinement products.

HOW TO ASSEMBLE A SKINCARE ROUTINE

Keeping this hierarchy of needs in mind should help simplify the complexities of building a skincare routine, whether from the ground up or from a foundation of products you're already using. We'll work our way up from the bottom, making sure your basics are in order before adding any of the treatment and refinement products you decide you'd like to try as well.

When it comes to building a skincare routine, following one simple rule will save you a lot of time, money, and potential skin problems: **only add one new item to your routine at a time**.

Skin can be finicky. Even if your skin isn't normally sensitive or acne-prone, the vast array of ingredients used in today's skincare products means the risk of irritation or reactions is always greater than zero. Introducing more than one product at a time will prevent you from knowing which product caused a reaction or breakout—in order to get to the bottom of the problem, you'd have to eliminate both products from your routine, wait for the reaction to subside or the breakout to heal, and then start over by introducing one of the new products at a time to see which one caused the issue.

So. Only add one new product at a time. Give it at least a week, and preferably two or three, to allow time for any slower-developing reactions to appear. If you experience any adverse effects, take the product out of your routine immediately (with the exception of purging from exfoliants, which we'll discuss in the treatment chapter). Wait until the irritation or breakout goes away before trying again with something else.

Don't get rid of the offending product right away, however. Make a note of the product and its full ingredients list. As you continue trying other products, you may begin to notice patterns: ingredients that always cause issues, for example, or product textures or consistencies that don't agree with your skin.

This will take longer than buying a prefab routine and slapping it all on your face right away. That's okay. In the long run, it will minimize problems and enable you to achieve the best results possible for your skin. It's worth the work.

TRACKING YOUR PROGRESS

As you begin painstakingly assembling your new skincare routine, you'll naturally want to make sure that each product you add, and your routine as a whole, are actually benefiting your skin. It may not sound like a huge issue—if your skin is improving, surely you'll see it in the mirror— but it often is.

Our brains are wonderfully skilled at showing us things that aren't there, or in this case, failing to show us things that are there. We get used to seeing ourselves in the mirror because we do every day. Incremental changes get logged as nothing of note by the brain. Time goes by. We continue to change. The brain continues to insist that we're the same as before. Most of us have either experienced this directly or known someone who's experienced it. For example, major weight loss that is barely registering, so that the person who is losing weight still perceives themselves as the same as before, or the other way around.

In just about any endeavor in which sustained effort produces incremental progress, many of us find ourselves constantly stressing about whether we're getting any better at all.

I have a good friend who's currently learning Mandarin Chinese. She's starting from scratch, with no prior knowledge of the language beyond watching subtitled Chinese dramas. She's putting hours into her language lessons and studying every day. In the short span of a month, she's learned enough vocabulary (both spoken and written) and internalized enough of our grammar to be able to put together many sentences on her own. She can read more than a few subtitles in the dramas she's watching. She's made incredible progress. And yet she struggles with feeling that she's not learning and not improving at all. From the outside, it's obvious she is, and rapidly. From the inside, it isn't.

The challenge our brains face in recognizing incremental improvement (again, in pretty much any endeavor) causes so much unnecessary discouragement. Most skincare products do not deliver overnight results. It takes time and consistency to produce real change. In the meantime, our face in the mirror looks the same as always to our flawed self-perception.

To get around this, I highly recommend a progress log. I do it for fitness and for creative projects, and I do it for skincare, too. Keeping track of what new products you're trying and when you started them will be useful for identifying any particularly problematic or particularly effective additions to your routine. On top of that, your skincare log can include progress photos.

Take a simple, straight-on, no makeup selfie once every week or two. Try to take it in the same location and with the same lighting each time. After a few weeks or a few months, you'll be able to see your skin's progress or lack thereof much more clearly. Having that more objective way of evaluating any changes to your skin can serve as a huge motivating factor.

I use a similar strategy for dealing with my general anxiety spirals. My anxiety often manifests as the conviction that my worst fear is about to come true or that nothing I do ever amounts to anything. To counteract this, I keep a journal entirely dedicated to all the times my fears didn't come to pass, as well as a log of my achievements and any milestones I hit. When I feel certain that a bad thing is going to happen, I look back at my journal. When I think I've never done anything good in my entire life and never will, I look at my achievements log. Over time, my anxiety spirals have significantly lessened in frequency and severity. I've taught myself through experience and repetition that those fears are not based in reality.

So it goes with your skincare. Keep track of what you're doing and for how long you've been doing it. Keep up with your progress photos. If you feel like you're doing everything right and nothing is changing, scroll through those, or put your oldest one side by side with your latest one. If your routine is consistent, the chances are good that you'll see much more improvement than you expected.

Of course, for improvement we need to go back to the basics and build up your routine. In the following chapters, we'll tackle this task one step at a time, following the structure laid out in my hierarchy of skincare needs.

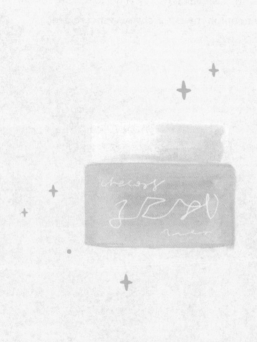

Chapter 3

SUSTENANCE: CLEANSING AND MOISTURIZING

Among all the exciting skincare community talk of things like actives, essences, serums, and sheet masks, it can be easy to overlook the basics of a good skincare routine. But without the foundation in place, the rest of the structure is doomed to collapse. Cleansing and moisturizing are the very basics of any skincare routine, keeping skin healthy and functioning as it should.

CLEANSING

Skincare products work best on clean skin. There's less to get in their way, so they penetrate and can therefore affect skin more thoroughly. If there's nothing foreign getting trapped in your skin, your risk of clogged pores also goes down. Cleansing, therefore, is absolutely critical to an effective skincare routine.

Luckily, of all the elements of a basic skincare routine, cleansing is the most intuitive. Skin gets dirty. Therefore, wash and make it clean. Done. Right?

Yeah. Kind of. But actually, no. There's a lot more to it than that, and a lot of room for error in the very basic mandate of cleansing. When it goes wrong, it can go terribly wrong, compromising your skin's health and appearance. When it goes right, however, it can work wonders. Simply changing my cleansing approach and finding the right products for me allowed me to cross multiple items off of the long list of grievances I had against my skin. And now I'll explain why.

Cleansing mistakes I have made over the years include washing my face with:

- A random bar soap
- Random body wash
- Random body wash applied with scrubby shower gloves
- Whatever random cleanser was on sale when I needed to buy more
- An exfoliating cleanser every single time I washed my face, so...twice a day

✦ Forgetting to remove my makeup beforehand

Inadequate cleansing leaves sweat, sebum, dirt, pollution, and/or makeup and sunscreen residue behind on skin, increasing the likelihood of clogged pores, acne, and even aging-accelerating free radical damage. Overcleansing or incorrectly cleansing is just as bad for your skin.

The Importance of Your Moisture Barrier

Remember how common skin conditions like dehydration, sensitization, and congestion could all be caused by a compromised moisture barrier? Let's discuss why.

The outermost layer of skin—called the stratum corneum,[1] the horny layer (my favorite term), the acid mantle, or simply the moisture barrier—exists to keep bacteria and other contaminants and irritants out of your skin and to hold moisture and the rest of your skin's contents in.

In order to achieve these objectives, the horny layer is structured to make skin as waterproof as possible. Think of it as a brick wall, where the bricks are flattened dead skin cells. The mortar that seals them together is made of your skin's naturally occurring lipids, including the lipids ceramide and sebum.

Stay with me here. While the layers of flattened dead skin cells are important to skin health, for the purposes of this cleansing discussion, we'll focus on the lipids. Lipids, like all other fatty substances, are hydrophobic: they repel water. All skin naturally loses its water over time in a process known as Trans Epidermal Water Loss (TEWL). In a healthy moisture barrier, however, those lipids help to minimize TEWL, allowing skin to remain hydrated, healthy, and glowing with moisture.

When we overcleanse, whether by using a cleansing product that's too harsh or by cleansing too frequently, we end up washing away too much of our horny layer's lipid content.[2] Imagine removing the mortar from a brick wall, and you can picture how this compromises the whole structure. Water can now escape your skin at an accelerated rate, leaving it looking dull and deflated and feeling tight and uncomfortable. Meanwhile, bacteria and irritants can enter through weak points, causing breakouts and reactions. It's not a good situation for your skin.

Cleansing without Consequences

I came of age in the 1990s. That was a very long time ago, but not so long ago that I don't remember my adolescent skincare practices. Those practices involved the harshest possible "anti-acne" face washes I could find at the drugstore. See, back in the olden days, it was believed that acne was caused by oily skin and that the cure for oily skin, and therefore acne, was to strip it of all its oils at every opportunity.

It didn't work. While I was lucky enough not to suffer from the more severe forms of acne, no Neutrogena, Clean & Clear, or Clinique cleanser I tried ever did a thing to prevent the sprouting of a pimple here, a couple there, enough to get remarked upon by family members during holiday gatherings. Overcleansing: not the solution. What *has* worked for me and for many others in today's skincare communities is a totally different approach to cleansing.

Instead of relying on violently overpowered single-step foam cleansers to get my skin clean, I've adopted the "double cleansing" method popularized by the Korean and Japanese beauty trends of the 2010s.

(There's some debate about whether double cleansing originated in the Korean or Japanese beauty industries. In my opinion, those debates are largely irrelevant, except to score nationalistic innovation points, so I'm not going to go there. There is also at least one major Western skincare influencer who claims to have invented double cleansing, but I am most *definitely* not going to go there. Just a bit of trivia for you.)

Double cleansing, as the name implies, is a two-step cleansing process. Generally, it involves using an emulsifying, oil-based first step cleanser to remove makeup and sunscreen, followed by a water-based second cleanser to wash away any remaining residue.

When done with the products appropriate to your skin's needs, double cleansing is a game changer. Foaming cleansers alone will either be too gentle to fully remove heavier or more long-wearing makeup and sunscreen products, or so harsh that they strip and damage your moisture barrier in the process. A good cleansing oil can break up and dissolve even waterproof products without drying your skin out, allowing you to finish the cleansing process with a much milder foaming cleanser. The result is sparkling clean but still healthy skin that's ready to receive the full benefits of the rest of your skincare routine.

We'll talk about the specific types of products you can use to double cleanse later in this chapter. Before we continue, though, let's clear up a few common misconceptions about double cleansing.

- **Double cleansing isn't** something you need to do twice a day. There's no need to use a cleansing oil in the morning unless you wake up with sunscreen and makeup still on from the day before (which you shouldn't if you already double cleansed the previous evening). Double cleansing is an evening-only step.

- **Double cleansing also isn't** something you need to do every evening. If you weren't wearing makeup or sunscreen that day, don't bother. In fact, on days when I've only worn very light or no makeup and a non-water-resistant sunscreen, I don't use a cleansing oil. I just swipe some cleansing water on my face with a cotton pad and proceed straight to my foaming cleanser.

- **Double cleansing also isn't** something you do with two different foaming cleansers or two consecutive applications of the same foaming cleanser. Doubling up on foaming cleansers tends to dry out skin even if the cleanser itself isn't overly harsh. Having a separate non-stripping makeup remover step like a cleansing oil or cleansing water is important.

Now, on to the products!

First Cleansers

Oil-based cleansers work remarkably well for removing even the most water-resistant makeup and sunscreen without drying skin out, which is why they're so common as first-step cleansers. In fact, some people simply use plain carrier oils like mineral oil or olive oil as their first step cleanser. I personally don't recommend that, however. Straight carrier oils are much more difficult to remove—the Oil Cleansing Method (OCM) typically involves scrubbing it off with a washcloth of some kind—and they're messier.

Instead, I use emulsifying cleansing oils and balms. These products contain some oil or combination of oils as their main ingredient but also add emulsifying agents. When massaged into dry skin (as in skin that you haven't first splashed with water), they feel and behave like oils. When you add water, however, they emulsify into a thin, milky foam that rinses off easily, taking your makeup and/or sunscreen with it. Easy and convenient.

Common Types of First Cleansers

Cleansing Oils and Cleansing Balms

The most common types of emulsifying, oil-based first cleansers you'll see are **cleansing oils** and **cleansing balms**. Cleansing oils are liquid and come in pump bottles. Cleansing balms are solid, with a soft waxy or sherbet-like consistency, and come in tubs. Both perform about the same, so whichever one you choose is down to your personal preference. I like to keep at least one cleansing balm handy in case of travel, since they don't spill or leak and don't count as liquids if you're traveling by air. To use, apply directly to a dry face. Massage gently for thirty seconds or so—if you have makeup on, you'll see it easily start smudging off. Wet hands and massage again to emulsify. Rinse, then follow with your second cleanser.

Cleansing Creams

You may also come across cleansing creams. These are more of a throwback to old-fashioned cold creams. They contain enough oil to massage away makeup and sunscreen but don't emulsify or rinse away easily. To use, massage them thoroughly over dry skin for about thirty seconds to a minute or until your makeup is visibly dissolved, then wipe off with a tissue or cloth. Wet your face and follow with your second cleanser. I don't love these, but they can come in handy if you're camping or in other situations where access to running water is limited.

You can also simply use a liquid makeup remover or makeup remover wipe as your first cleanser, though I find this tends to be harsher on skin than using a cleansing oil or balm, due to the extra scrubbing you need to do with a cotton pad, tissue, or the wipe itself. As I've mentioned before, however, I do like cleansing waters for a very light first cleanse step. They aren't as harsh, and if my cotton pad is saturated well, it doesn't take much scrubbing.

How to Choose a First Cleanser

Since first cleansers are wash-off products whose sole purpose is to clean your skin and then go away, rather than to stay on your skin and produce a longer-term effect, there's generally little need to be choosy about them. They don't have to be fancy and they don't need to include any active ingredients or exotic extracts that may drive up their price. As long as the one you choose cleanses well, doesn't break you out or irritate your skin, and doesn't break your budget, you're good to go. Here's a quick recap:

- **Cleansing oils** and **cleansing balms** are your most common choices for first cleansers. Both will lift off and break up makeup and sunscreen, then emulsify and rinse away with water.

- **Cleansing creams** remove makeup and sunscreen in a similar fashion as cleansing oils and balms, but since they don't emulsify with water and must be wiped off, can be less convenient for daily use. They do come in handy in situations where running water is limited, however.

- **Makeup removers** and **makeup remover wipes** generally work fine for the first cleansing step but are harsher on skin than the above options.

First cleansers *do* go on your skin, so here are some tips to keep in mind in case you aren't yet familiar with your skin's quirks.

- If your skin is prone to clogged pores or acne, but you're not sure what ingredients exacerbate these issues, you may want to avoid products that contain olive oil or coconut oil. These oils draw lots of praise from the natural-is-better crowd, but many people find them clogging and comedogenic. Mineral oil is generally a safer bet. The molecules are too large to penetrate skin, and although the natural-is-better crowd fears it due to the fact that it's a byproduct of crude oil refinement, cosmetic grade mineral oil has been deemed perfectly safe for human use for decades.

If your skin is sensitive, but you're not sure what ingredients irritate it, try to avoid products that contain fragrance, including fragrant essential oils like lavender, bergamot, orange, limonene, or linalool. These are common triggers for sensitive skin reactions.

Can "Non-Comedogenic" Products Break Me Out?

As you shop for your skincare, you'll see the terms "comedogenic" and "non-comedogenic" on plenty of product labels. "Comedogenic" means that the ingredient is known, according to some very flawed and limited tests,[3] to cause acne. Some ingredients, like olive oil and coconut oil, are considered more likely to be comedogenic than others. This doesn't mean that every "comedogenic" ingredient must be avoided. Everyone's skin is different; not everyone will break out due to a comedogenic ingredient, and some people may break out due to ingredients generally considered non-comedogenic. And the term "non-comedogenic" on a product label means next to nothing. The use of this term isn't regulated at all and does not constitute a promise that you won't break out. The best thing you can do for your skin is to pay attention to your own reactions to products, gradually developing a better understanding of what does and doesn't work for *you*.

Second Cleansers

Although second cleansers, like first cleansers, are just wash-off products that aren't expected to add any long-term effects besides getting skin clean, I find that one's choice of second cleanser makes a much bigger difference to skin.

It goes back to the moisture barrier. While barrier health can be affected by other steps in a skincare routine, it's often the foaming cleanser that makes or breaks its overall structure and function, and therefore your skin's health and appearance. Be picky about your second cleanser. It matters much more than you may expect.

Cleansers work by grabbing loose particles on your skin and hanging on to them as the cleanser is rinsed away. Some cleansers are gentle enough to only latch on to the looser particles, like dirt and excess sebum. Others operate by essentially snatching everything that isn't solidly nailed down, including things your skin should hold on to, like the all-important naturally occurring lipids in your skin's moisture barrier.

Why Does the pH of My Cleanser Matter?

The pH of a healthy moisture barrier usually falls somewhere between 4.5 and 6, which is mildly acidic. It's the acidity of this part of the skin that helps make it an inhospitable environment for bacteria, one of the ways that the horny layer can prevent breakouts.

When you use a cleanser whose pH is too high, two things happen. One, the excessively alkaline pH weakens and disrupts the acid mantle. And two, thanks to that weakening effect, the cleansing agents in your high pH cleanser are able to grab and make off with more of your skin's natural lipids, stripping it of its protection against TEWL and external irritants. While a low pH doesn't guarantee a perfectly gentle cleanser, a high pH cleanser is much more likely to damage skin.[4]

To recover and maintain a healthy moisture barrier, choose a foaming cleanser at a barrier-friendly pH: lower than 7 at least. Some purists cite pH 5.5 as their cutoff.

Unfortunately, there are many more alkaline cleansers on the market than there are acidic ones. According to some friends of mine at major cosmetics brands, high pH cleansers are popular because they provide a "squeaky clean" effect, which communicates to the consumer that the cleanser really did clean their skin. It did—that's not the problem. The problem is that the cleanser cleansed too well. That squeaking is a sign that your acid mantle has lost a significant amount of its lipids.

The main obstacle to identifying good, pH-appropriate cleansers for your skin is the unwillingness of many brands to put the pH of their products on their product labels. Luckily for the modern skincare enthusiast, however, many bloggers have taken to purchasing pH testing strips and publishing the results of their own cleanser tests. If a particular cleanser catches your eye, Google its pH. You may find the answer. Alternatively, you can always purchase litmus strips and test cleansers yourself.

Some brands market their cleansers as "pH balanced." Much like the term "non-comedogenic," "pH balanced" is an unregulated and therefore almost meaningless term. Generally, though, a "pH balanced" cleanser will have a pH of around 7, making it a decent place to start.

In addition to pH, the type of surfactants (foaming/cleansing agents) each cleanser uses will affect its relative gentleness or harshness. Keep that in mind as you choose a second cleanser.

Common Cleansing Agents in Second Cleansers

The harshest cleansers will contain **some kind of fat or oil (myristic, palmitic, and lauric acids are common)** and a strong base, typically either **sodium hydroxide or**

potassium hydroxide, both of which have a very high pH. The reaction between the fat or oil and the sodium or potassium hydroxide is called saponification. It produces soap, which I find far too stripping and alkaline for facial skin. I don't recommend true soaps for anyone's face, no matter how oily their skin is.

Moving down the list from most stripping to most gentle, **sodium lauryl sulfate** (SLS) doesn't appear in as many facial cleansers as it once did, due to the common perception of its harshness as a cleansing agent. In a high pH cleanser, I do find SLS too stripping. With that being said, I have used at least a couple of low pH cleansers that contained SLS and found those cleansers to be fine.

Sodium laureth sulfate (SLES) is a slightly milder surfactant that performs similarly to SLS for me. I consider SLS and SLES in a neutral to low pH cleanser to be generally fine for oily and normal skin.

For drier and/or more sensitive skin, **cocamidylpropyl betaine**, a.k.a. **coco betaine**, tends to work better. Milder than SLES, it presents less risk of dryness. Coco betaine generally foams less than SLS or SLES, which may make it less satisfying to use if you're used to highly foamy cleansers, though they're still effective.

Common Types of Second Cleansers

Foaming Cleansers

The most common type of second cleanser you'll encounter is the **foaming cleanser**. These are the ones we're all familiar with. The relative gentleness of a foaming cleanser will depend largely on its pH and the surfactants it uses[5], with high pH, soap- or SLS-based cleansers being most harsh and low pH, coco betaine-based cleansers offering milder cleansing action. To use, mix the cleanser with water in your hand to create a foam, then massage over your face for thirty seconds or so and rinse thoroughly.

Alternatively, some foaming cleansers come packaged with a foaming pump that agitates the product with air when the pump is pressed down, dispensing a puff of mousse-like foam. This is a nice workaround for the less-foamy coco betaine cleansers, providing a nice foam without sacrificing gentleness. You'll recognize foaming pumps by the thicker base of the pump lid.

Gel Cleansers

Gel cleansers are typically gentler than foaming cleansers, due to their lack of highly foaming surfactants. They produce little to no lather when mixed with water and are a good choice for skin that's too dry or sensitive for even the mildest foaming cleansers. To use, dispense onto hands and massage gently over your face for thirty seconds, then rinse thoroughly.

Cleansing Waters/Micellar Waters

Within the "water-based cleanser" category, you'll also find **cleansing waters** and **micellar waters**. These are watery, non-foaming liquids that contain a low concentration of surfactants. I think of these as first step makeup removers, particularly for light makeup and/or non-water resistant sunscreens. To use, saturate a cotton pad and lightly swipe over face. Try not to rub or scrub too much.

How to Choose Your Second Cleanser

Now that you have a clearer sense of the importance of cleanser pH, the relative harshness of the most common surfactants, and the differences between the types of second cleansers, you should have a better idea of what kind of cleanser to look for. As a quick recap:

- Look for a cleanser at a pH of 7 or below to preserve the integrity of your moisture barrier.

- If your skin is oily or normal, your range of choices is fairly broad: foaming cleansers with SLS, SLES, or coco betaine all stand a good chance of working out for you.
- If your skin is more dry or sensitive, the safest options will be gel cleansers with coco betaine.

Don't worry about the special ingredients or extraordinary claims with which some cleansers are marketed. Since these are wash-off products, it's unlikely that they will treat acne, address signs of aging, or otherwise target specific skin issues. The function of a cleanser is to cleanse, so make that your main priority when choosing one.

How to Minimize Your Starting Costs

Assembling a skincare routine requires a certain amount of trial and error for pretty much everyone. A product may sound great for you in theory but end up flopping for a number of reasons—unexpected reactions, an unpleasant texture or scent, or simple failure to perform its intended function.

To minimize your expense and waste, seek out sample and travel-sized products wherever you can. Many brands put out mini sizes of new or popular products or offer gift sets with several different mini products. Per ounce, the prices tend to be higher than they would be for the same product in full size, but if you suspect you'll need to try a few products before finding the right one, grabbing several different travel sizes could be more economical.

MOISTURIZING

The value of the most fundamental steps in your skincare routine lies in their ability to maintain an ideal balance of oil and water in your skin so that it can most effectively retain moisture and repel contaminants. As we've seen, cleansing can make or break your skin's ability to do so. Moisturizing is just as important.

Moisturizer, as the name implies, exists to add extra moisture to your skin. Even the healthiest skin will lose water throughout the day or night, and as we get older, our skin's ability to hang on to water naturally decreases. Think of moisturizer as not only a means of adding more moisture, but also as a secondary barrier for your skin, supporting its primary barrier function. Moisturizer can also smooth the surface of your skin, giving it a more even-textured appearance.

Types of Moisturizing Ingredients

Back in *my day*, moisturizers came in a pretty limited selection. There were day creams, night creams, and lotions. These days, there are creams, day creams, night creams, water drop creams, gels, gel creams, lotions, and emulsions. Some have tint. Some have SPF. Some have actives like retinol or vitamin C. We have a lot of choices. Narrowing those choices down to the ones that will work best for your skin will take some understanding of what goes into them.

Among the many ingredients you'll find in moisturizers are the ingredients that actually add moisture to your skin. Roughly, these fall into three categories: humectants, emollients, and occlusives. Most moisturizers will contain some mix of two or all three types; the ratios between them are what differentiate the products.

Humectants

Humectants are ingredients that bind to water and carry it into the epidermis, adding hydration to the skin. They may also draw water up from deeper layers of the skin to more thoroughly hydrate near the surface. A hydrating moisturizer gives temporarily plumper and firmer skin, and since skin, like any other organ in the body, is healthiest when well hydrated, humectants may also help skin heal, regenerate, and function at its best. The most common humectants you'll find are **glycerin** and various forms of **hyaluronic acid**, including **sodium hyaluronate** and **hydrolyzed hyaluronic acid**.

Hyaluronic acid is a particularly interesting ingredient due to the fact that several forms of it appear in skincare. The forms of hyaluronic acid are differentiated by their molecular weight: the smaller the molecule, the deeper it can penetrate into skin. There is a trade-off to this, however. Generally, the higher molecular weights of hyaluronic acid can bind more water for longer, while the lower molecular weight hyaluronic acids can get deeper into skin but hold less water for less time. I like hydrating products that contain a mix of different hyaluronic acids so my skin can receive the best of all worlds.

Hyaluronic acid occurs naturally in our bodies. Our production of it decreases as we age, making supplementing it with topical humectants more important to skin health and appearance as we get older.

Some other common humectants you'll find in skincare are glycols, like **propylene glycol** and **butylene glycol**; **sorbitol**; **sodium PCA**; **allantoin**; **panthenol**; **sodium lactate**; **urea**; and alpha hydroxy acids like **lactic acid** and **glycolic acid**. A number of natural ingredients contain humectant properties as well—**honey** and **snail mucin**, a.k.a. **snail secretion filtrate**, are two of my favorites.

Myth: Humectants Are Bad for Skin in Dry Weather

You may hear people claim that you shouldn't use humectant-heavy products in very arid conditions. According to this myth, if the air around you is too dry, the humectants will suck the water right out of your skin and into the air. This isn't true. You will still experience your normal rate of TEWL, but not an accelerated one.

The reason people perceive hydrating products to be drying in dry conditions is simply because of the fact that skin will feel dryer in dry conditions to begin with, and the sensation of product evaporating from the surface of skin can be mistaken for the skin itself drying out more than normal. To prevent this sensation, simply make sure to use a moisturizer with enough emollient and occlusive properties to slow down TEWL.

Emollients and Occlusives

Let's return for a moment to earlier in this chapter, where we envisioned the stratum corneum as a brick and mortar structure of flattened dead skin cells held together by lipids. At a microscopic level, the very top layer of this structure will not be perfectly smooth. There are tiny cracks and crevices between the cells and where some lipids are missing.

Emollients are moisturizing ingredients, typically fatty, whose molecular size allows them to fill in those cracks and crevices. This enables them to reinforce the barrier structure of skin and deliver a softer and more supple overall texture.

Like humectants, some emollients used in skincare are produced naturally by our skin, but production often declines as we get older. Some emollients you'll see in skincare are **ceramides**, **lanolin**, **caprylic/capric triglyceride**, **squalane**, **squalene**, **cetyl alcohol**, **cetearyl alcohol**, **beeswax**, **mineral oil**, and **petrolatum**. Many plant oils and butters are also emollient, among them **olive** and **coconut oils** and **shea and coconut butters**.

When used in high enough concentrations or applied generously enough to skin, emollient moisturizing ingredients also have an occlusive effect, meaning that they form a protective layer on top of skin to hold hydration in. While nothing can fully halt water loss from even healthy skin, occlusive moisturizers can significantly reduce it. For this purpose, emollient ingredients of larger molecular sizes are most effective. If you need a very occlusive product, look for mineral oil- or petrolatum-based moisturizers. In fact, some people swear by Vaseline as their nighttime moisturizer.

How to Read An Ingredients List

Since the balance of humectant and emollient ingredients in a moisturizer will determine its moisturizing properties and suitability for your skin's needs, now is a good time to learn the basics of reading an ingredients list.

Different countries have different regulations about how ingredients must be listed on a product's label, but at the time of this book's publication, the US, the EU, South Korea, Taiwan, and Japan require all ingredients present in concentrations of greater than 1 percent of the total product volume to be shown in descending order from the highest concentration down. In other words, whatever ingredient is present in the greatest amount will be the first ingredient on the list, followed by the ingredient present in the second greatest amount, then the third, and so on.

In the vast majority of products, the first five or so ingredients will be the ones that take up the bulk of the product's volume, so pay special attention to those ingredients, and you'll get a rough idea of the product's humectant and emollient balance. It's not a perfect system, since you won't know the exact concentrations, but in general, it will help you identify products more suited to your needs.

Types of Moisturizers

Moisturizers are among the most common and widely used skincare products, and the global cosmetics industry caters to consumers with a staggering array of moisturizer varieties, some more suitable to certain skin types than others. Outliers that don't perform as their name suggests do exist, but in general, you can narrow down your initial moisturizer selection by understanding what to expect from the different types. To simplify this process, I've broken them down here according to the skin types they typically work best for.

Dry to Very Dry Skin

Moisturizers that contain high amounts of emollient ingredients work best for dry to very dry skin, since the added emollients help compensate for the underproduction of natural oils that characterizes dry skin.

Facial Oils

If your skin underproduces oils, then theoretically, it makes sense to reach for an oil to lubricate it. Facial oils are liquid moisturizers meant to do just that. Some are simply single oils, like squalene or rosehip. Others are blends of several different oils. The lightest blends may also contain some aqueous and humectant ingredients, resulting in a less oily and more serum-like consistency and finish. Most brands market facial oils not only for their moisturizing qualities, but also for whatever secondary benefits the oils in question may provide, such as antioxidant content to delay visible skin aging.

While many people swear by the use of a facial oil for dry skin, others find these products challenging to use. They can leave an unpleasant oily film on top of skin. Some find that oils rub off more easily than other types of moisturizers. And even "hydrating" oil blends often fail to provide enough aqueous and humectant content to hydrate skin that lacks water as well as oil. Still, I find it worthwhile to have at least one oil on hand for mixing into other products on days when my skin needs more richness than my regular moisturizers provide.

Balms

Like facial oils, balm-type moisturizers can excel at providing emollient and occlusive moisture to shore up the outer surface of dry skin. Often made with a high concentration of petrolatum for a softer consistency or beeswax or lanolin for a more waxy consistency, balms form a strongly occlusive layer on the skin to hold moisture in.

Like facial oils, balm moisturizers are often lacking in the hydration department, since the bulk of the product must be emollient in order to achieve the right consistency. They are often more pleasant to use than oils, however, especially when made to dry down to a soft and non-greasy finish. In my experience, they also stick around longer on skin than many oils do.

All Skin Types

Creams, Lotions, and Emulsions

The huge variety of water to oil ratios and subsequent consistencies and finishes in creams means that just about any skin type can find a cream appropriate for their moisture needs, with some containing higher amounts of emollient oils to benefit dry skin and others achieving a lighter consistency and more hydrating effect by emphasizing humectants and silicones in their ingredients. Heavier creams often work well for skin that is both dry and dehydrated, since they deliver more humectant content than oils or balms. Lotions and emulsions typically provide similar moisture levels as creams, but in a softer liquid format.

Day Creams vs. Night Creams

While I prefer a lighter moisturizer for day and a heavier one at night, not everyone needs a separate day and night cream.

Generally, moisturizers marketed as "day creams" contain SPF. While this may sound like a great way to combine two important steps into one, the actual protection of a day cream is often less than ideal (we'll discuss why in detail in the next chapter). "Night creams," meanwhile, tend to be heavier and often contain anti-aging ingredients as well as moisturizing ones.

Any moisturizer can be used at any time of day, depending on your individual skin needs. Don't take a product's name as a rule—just choose one that feels right for your skin, no matter what time of day it's "supposed" to be used.

Normal Skin

Moisturizers with a fairly even balance of humectant and emollient ingredients tend to work well for normal skin, providing some extra hydration and guarding against TEWL without feeling too heavy.

Gel Creams

The water and humectant content in gel creams tends to be higher compared to its fatty content than in traditional cream moisturizers, and gel creams often use more silicones than oils or plant butters for their emollient content. This makes them more lightweight than creams, though with the ability to provide a significant amount of moisture. Skin that is dehydrated but not too dry often does well with gel cream moisturizers.

Oily Skin

Skin that already overproduces oils doesn't need much extra in the way of emollient moisture but often still benefits from added hydration and texture smoothing.

Gel Moisturizers

Gel moisturizers are heavily water- and humectant-based, relying largely on some light silicone content to create a nearly imperceptible emollient film over the surface of skin. This allows them to hydrate and soften oily skin without adding greasiness. Some gel moisturizers also contain notable alcohol content, which can aid in temporarily reducing oiliness on skin.

Water Drop Creams

While gimmicky, these can be fun! Water drop creams are very lightweight moisturizers whose formulation allows them to break up into visible beads of liquid on skin before absorbing. They add a refreshing sensation and weightless hydration for normal to oily skin.

Are Special Ingredients in Moisturizers Worth It?

Many brands market their moisturizers as multipurpose. As I mentioned earlier, some contain SPF, while others offer retinol or vitamin C to support anti-aging claims. Still others contain ingredients to address acne or calm sensitivity. These added claims help differentiate the moisturizers from competing products and provide justification for higher prices, but are they worth it?

If you don't intend to extend your skincare routine further than cleansing and moisturizing, but you would like to achieve improvements in your skin beyond simply maintaining its cleanliness and moisture levels, then moisturizers with added effects may be better than nothing, provided the moisturizers actually contain an effective amount of the special ingredients featured.

Effective concentrations are the sticking point. In my experience, very few products marketed as multipurpose actually fulfill any of their secondary purposes well. Formulating a moisturizer with the expected consistency, moisturizing effect, and "skinfeel" requires specific ratios of water, humectants, emollients, and the emulsifiers needed to bind the aqueous and fatty ingredients together into a pleasant and uniform whole. This often leaves little room for the incorporation of effective concentrations of other ingredients. Again, however, if you really don't want to add more products to your skincare routine, something may be better than nothing.

Are Eye Creams Worth It?

I don't think eye cream will ever stop generating mild controversy in skincare circles. On one side sit the people who consider eye creams a scam, just heavy moisturizer packaged in smaller jars with a different name, marked up to a higher cost per ounce than their full-face equivalents in larger containers. On the other side sit people who swear by this or that eye cream and would never think of putting a regular face cream around their eyes.

The truth, in my opinion, lies somewhere in the middle. If taken out of their packaging, most eye creams *are* indistinguishable from regular face creams, and few do anything special. Some exceptions do exist for me—I can think of three eye creams I've used over the years that have significantly tightened and firmed the skin around my eyes. But "special properties for the eye area" isn't the only consideration when it comes to choosing a moisturizer for this part of the face.

The skin around our eyes tends to be drier and thinner than the skin on the rest of our face and becomes even more so as we age. It loses elasticity more rapidly, which is a concern for people who want to delay the visible aging process. And it happens to surround our actual eyes, which are usually more sensitive to potential irritants like alcohol and fragrance than our faces. Because of these considerations, many of us prefer a separate cream for our eyes that provides more moisture, a stronger firming effect, and fewer potential irritants than the moisturizers we like to use on our faces.

Do *you* need a separate eye cream? As with every other step in your skincare routine, that's up to you. If you're unsure, simply use the moisturizer you've chosen for your face around your eyes for a while and see how you like it. If you aren't satisfied with the effects of your facial moisturizer around your eyes, consider looking for a separate eye cream. There aren't any eye-specific ingredients to look out for, so focus on finding one that adds whatever your face cream is missing when you put it around your eyes, such as a greater emphasis on emollient moisture for very dry eyelids or higher water and humectant content for dehydrated, crepey skin.

THE POWER OF A DAILY SKINCARE ROUTINE

I've written before and sometimes at length about how skincare has become a life-changing method for managing my depression. My story resonates with most people who read it, but inevitably I'll get at least a few doubters who wonder how something so trivial could produce such a profound effect.

I struggled with Major Depressive Disorder for over a decade before I finally stumbled across a path out of the long, deep depressive episodes. As you might have guessed, that path involved skincare.

When my depressive episodes hit, they take away nearly all my motivation to do anything beyond what's necessary for basic survival. A thick cloud of negativity settles over all of my thoughts and ideas; my internal monologue becomes an endless repetition of *What's the point? It's not like anything ever improves anyway.*

I have plans. I've always had plans, some of them big plans. Really big ones, especially when I was younger.

However, most of those plans fizzled out because I couldn't bring myself to take the small steps needed to execute them. The small steps loomed huge in my mind, the goal looked impossibly distant, and none of the potential rewards seemed worth the Herculean effort of slogging through the necessary work to get there. Depression tricked me into thinking that anything worth doing would be impossibly hard and therefore pointless to attempt.

Skincare slipped past the barriers put up by my depressive thinking precisely because it is so "trivial." It piggybacked on a task I could already manage to do most of the time. If I was already in the shower, I wouldn't overthink taking the extra thirty seconds to wash my face. If I was already washing my face, using a more carefully chosen cleanser required no extra effort. And if I'd already washed my face, I might as well put moisturizer on afterwards, especially since if I didn't, my skin might feel tight and uncomfortable.

Cleansing and moisturizing easily became a small extra daily (well, more or less daily) routine for me, and that routine blossomed from there. The almost immediate improvement I saw in my skin once I started using products that suited it served as a reward and motivation to keep going. Choosing products that provided some extra entertainment value—whether through charming packaging, pleasing scents and textures, or an interesting ingredient story—added enjoyment to the routine. I found myself looking forward to washing my face. It became a fun little daily interlude, something that got me up and into the bathroom in the morning and something to look forward to at the end of the day.

I realized after some time that I was doing something deeper for myself, too. The act of taking care of my skin at the beginning and the end of the day had become a way of telling myself that I have value and deserve care. With repetition, that subconscious message managed to penetrate layers of apathy and self-doubt. It became my truth.

It not only became my truth, but a gateway into a whole world of rewarding habits that have given me the sense of control over my life that I lacked for years. During depressive slumps, I used to let everything slide: work, housework, self-care. The guilt I felt over letting myself and my life fall into disarray would then worsen the depression, creating a vicious cycle of neglect worsened by the feelings of guilt and hopelessness brought on the results of that neglect.

While I still experience those slumps (and most likely always will), they no longer have the power to prevent me from taking care of my surroundings or myself. I might let things slip for one or two days—in skincare terms, that mostly means that I might not wash my face one day because I don't intend to leave the house therefore don't need to apply sunscreen anyway. But I find it much easier to get back on the horse now than before, both with skincare and the other habits I've developed.

These days, I've come to appreciate the benefits of routine in more ways than just skincare. I have my morning bed-making routine, my nightly dishwashing and general tidying routine, my weekly housecleaning routine, and my regular yoga and exercise routines. But my skincare routine started it all. Not bad for a few minutes of face washing and moisturizing a day.

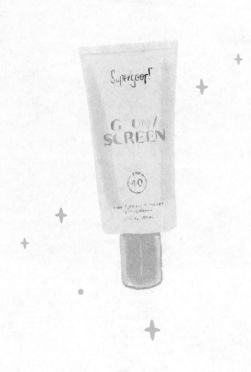

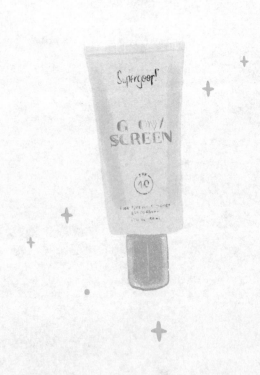

Chapter 4

PROTECTION: SUNSCREENS

None of us exists in a vacuum. We leave our homes regularly to work, to shop, socialize, and *live*. And in the course of our daily existence, we expose our skin to external factors that affect its health and appearance. We can't avoid most of these risks, but we can minimize them.

For both health and beauty purposes, the sun poses the greatest threat to our skin. As good as it feels, as life-giving as it is to plants, as important as it is for human mental health and vitamin D production, the simple fact of the matter is that sunlight is radiation, and radiation is hazardous to health.

The sun (and tanning beds) emit UV radiation, which greatly increases the risk of skin cancer. According to the International Agency for Research on Cancer, a part of the World Health Organization, UV radiation, including both natural sunlight and the light produced by the bulbs used in artificial tanning beds, is carcinogenic.[6] This is most likely due to the ability of certain types of UV radiation to alter DNA at the molecular level, leading to cancerous mutations. The more sun exposure a person receives throughout their life, the higher their chances of developing skin cancer.

As if that weren't enough to hammer home the risks of unprotected sun exposure, research also shows that UV radiation causes the vast majority of visible, extrinsic skin aging.[7]

Researchers generally separate visible skin aging into two distinct categories. **Intrinsic skin aging** refers to largely unavoidable, genetically determined changes in skin over time. The rate at which these changes happen and the specific ways they manifest will depend on our ethnicity and personal genetics.

No matter what we do, our skin will most likely lose some elasticity and develop some fine wrinkles over time. Our skin may become paler, thinner, and drier. If we've taken consistent care of it over the course of our lives, these effects may not become especially apparent until we hit our fifties and sixties, and we can mitigate the appearance of many of these effects with skincare, but we can't prevent them.

Extrinsic skin aging, on the other hand, is almost entirely preventable, since it's caused by external, lifestyle factors: primarily smoking and sun exposure.

If you go back and look at my description of intrinsic skin aging, you'll most likely think, *Well, that isn't too extreme.* And you'd be right. When we visualize women whom we describe as "aging well," we don't typically mean their seventy-year-old face is as firm as that of a thirty-year-old's and entirely free of wrinkles. We mean that while we can see their age in the increased laxity and pallor of their skin, it's really not that dramatic.

The effects of the inexorable forward march of time on our skin are unavoidable but can be lessened. The effects of sun and smoking, on the other hand...

Intrinsic skin aging is slow and subtle. **Extrinsic skin aging** caused by UV radiation can be rapid and profound. Collagen and elastin break down, leading to deep wrinkles and sagging. Discoloration and irregular pigmentation replace skin's youthful translucency and glow; skin texture becomes leathery. Enlarged, visible blood vessels near the surface of skin are another sign of photodamage, as well as chronic inflammation.

Severely UV-damaged skin is unmistakable once you recognize it, and these signs of UV damage can appear very early in life—late teens and early twenties for some, even.

If you're at all like me, you may have spent much of your youth blithely ignoring any parental attempts to get you to put on sunscreen before going to the pool or beach, or spending a day outdoors with friends. If you're at all like me, you may have started to heed those warnings at some point in your twenties, but mistook a tiny dab of SPF 15 face lotion for proper sun protection. If you're at all like me, you ended up with hyperpigmentation and textural changes at a relatively young age as a result of your early carelessness.

And that's okay. The damage *is*, at least to some extent, reversible. But first we must stop further damage from occurring.

SUNSCREEN

The most powerful tool in any skincare routine is sunscreen. Is your main skincare goal to delay or address

the visible signs of skin aging? You need sunscreen.
Is your main skincare goal to fade hyperpigmentation
for a more even skin tone? You need sunscreen. Is your
main skincare goal to minimize breakouts? You still need
sunscreen if you want to prevent the dark spots that
pimples can leave behind. Is your main skincare goal to
avoid developing skin cancer? You one hundred percent
definitely need sunscreen, unless you plan to adopt a
vampire schedule and never encounter the sun.

The thing is, any old SPF product, used any old way, won't
cut it. SPF in your foundation won't cut it. A tiny dab of
SPF 15 face lotion won't cut it.

According to the Skin Cancer Foundation, a sunscreen's
sun protection factor (SPF) indicates how long UVB
radiation would take to cause sunburn, compared to the
time it would take for you to burn without it.[8] So if your
skin generally burns after an hour in the sun, SPF 15
sunscreen will theoretically allow you to spend 15 hours
in the sun without burning…as long as you're using it
generously all over exposed skin and reapplying it after
a couple of hours of sun exposure or after getting wet
or sweaty.

Other cosmetic chemistry experts disagree with the "SPF rating indicates how much longer it will take for your skin to burn than without sunscreen" interpretation. Instead, these experts explain that SPF values indicate the percentage of UVB radiation absorbed by the product. This way of looking at it helps prevent people from going too long without reapplying sunscreen and puts the numbers into clearer perspective.

SPF: How High is High Enough?

Go into the sunscreen aisle of just about any drugstore, and you'll see a range of available SPFs—typically from as low as SPF 8 to as high as SPF 100. How high is high enough?

The Skin Cancer Foundation recommends applying broad spectrum sunscreen with a minimum of SPF 15 generously every day and upgrading to a broad spectrum, water-resistant sunscreen with a minimum of SPF 30 for swimming and other "extended outdoor activity." That is a minimum recommendation, however. You may find that your skin continues to redden or develop dark spots or other obvious signs of sun damage unless you increase your SPF. Personally, I only use sunscreens with an SPF of 45 or above and a rating of PA+++ or higher for everyday.

As the SPF of a sunscreen product increases, its cosmetic elegance often decreases. Higher SPF formulations are more likely to look chalky or feel heavy, due to the higher concentrations of UV filters they contain, especially if they contain physical filters. Ultimately, I recommend choosing the highest protection sunscreen you can find *that you can comfortably wear in the recommended quantities.* Being able to actually use the product properly is key to benefiting from it.

The SPF values on sunscreen products of any type—whether lotion, cream, spray, or powder—are determined by measuring the sunscreen's protection against UVB radiation when the product is applied on skin at a thickness of 2mg/sq cm[9]. That works out to roughly a quarter of a teaspoon for your face alone, and another quarter of a teaspoon for your neck and upper chest. The less you apply, the less protection you'll get. For the most reliable protection against sun damage, it's best to apply the full amount.

SPF is just the beginning, though. SPF denotes the protection the product will give against shorter wavelength UVB radiation. UVB radiation is responsible for sunburns and most skin cancers, according to the American Cancer Society. So SPF *is* critical for the basic health of your skin. If you want to delay visible skin aging and/or prevent and fade dark spots, however, you need to look for strong UVA protection as well. This is where US-made sunscreens fall short.

UVA radiation has a longer wavelength than UVB. UVB radiation damages the upper layers of skin; UVA radiation penetrates more deeply, causing DNA damage at the inner layers of skin.[10] UVA radiation leads to tanning (which is a defensive response to sun damage), dark spots, and the drastic and visible extrinsic skin aging that we discussed in the previous section.

In the US, UVA protection is denoted simply by the label "broad spectrum," which doesn't mean much. A broad spectrum sunscreen might provide significant UVA protection, or it might only provide the minimum effective UVA protection needed to earn the broad spectrum designation.

Korean and Japanese sunscreen labeling offers more insight into the UVA protection a product delivers by using PA ratings, which denote the strength of UVA protection a product provides, with PA+ being the lowest and PA++++ being the highest allowed at the time of this book's publication.

Types of UV Filters

Broadly, sunscreens are grouped into two main categories according to the type of UV filters they contain: "physical" (a.k.a. mineral or inorganic) and "chemical" (a.k.a. organic), although some sunscreens utilize both "physical" and "chemical" UV filters in a single product.

Before we get into the differences between those, as well as their advantages and disadvantages, let's talk for a minute about terminology. The terms "physical" and "chemical" are both misnomers, and the connotations of "chemical" in particular have enabled copious amounts of misinformation and fearmongering to spread, sometimes scaring people off from trying products that could be extremely well suited to their needs.

Everything is a chemical. "Chemical" simply means a substance made out of matter. Water is a chemical. Air is made of chemicals. The most wholesome organic non-GMO apple ever grown is also made out of chemicals—as are we. In modern culture, however, the term "chemical" has taken on connotations of artificiality. "Chemicals" are often juxtaposed against natural substances; you can see this taking place on cosmetics labels all over the beauty aisles of your local drugstores, despite the fact that the naturally derived ingredients such labeling touts are also made of chemicals.

This marketing is remarkably effective. There's an implied claim behind it: that what is natural is inherently better than what is artificial or synthetic. Whether "better" means "safer" or "more potent" depends on the exact product being marketed. Just know, before we go any farther, that the idea that "natural is better" is absolutely, objectively untrue. Botulism, arsenic, cyanide, rattlesnake poison, poison ivy, poison oak, deadly puffer fish, and the gympie gympie bush, a.k.a. the "suicide plant," are all natural. None of those are safe for humans. Meanwhile, synthetic cosmetic ingredients are standardized for purity and effectiveness and tested for safety.

Point being, chemical sunscreens often get a bad reputation, almost entirely based on their name. And while some chemical UV filters are unsuitable for some people's skin, they are not, across the board, less safe or less effective than physical filters.

Which is also a misnomer.

While the term "physical" sunscreen implies that physical filters work by creating a physical barrier against UV radiation (picture the chalky layers of zinc oxide on the noses of surfers and lifeguards), this is actually true of both physical and chemical sunscreens. No matter which type of UV filter it uses, a sunscreen product must form an even film—a physical barrier of sorts—over skin to provide optimal protection.

It's also often believed that physical UV filters work by physically reflecting UV radiation, deflecting those pesky photons before they can penetrate skin. In fact, physical and chemical UV filters both work primarily by absorbing UV rays and converting their energy to heat.

Barring personal sensitivities to specific ingredients, the functional differences between "physical" and "chemical" sunscreens are far less significant than how they are sometimes presented. There are some differences, however, so let's take a look at those.

Physical/Mineral/Inorganic UV Filters

There are only two physical UV filters currently in use: **zinc oxide** and **titanium dioxide**. These are produced by processing naturally occurring mineral sources of zinc or titanium, hence the alternative "mineral sunscreen" moniker. Because zinc oxide and titanium dioxide lack carbon-hydrogen bonds, they are also classified as "inorganic" compounds.

When we think of the stereotypical thick, chalky, oily-feeling sunscreen, the kind that puts us off of wearing sunscreen every day, what we're typically thinking of are physical sunscreens. Titanium dioxide in particular tends to leave a very noticeable white cast, though zinc oxide often does as well. Zinc oxide is a common active ingredient in diaper creams, which should give you an idea of how that ingredient tends to look. Both filters generally result in less cosmetically elegant formulations than "chemical"/organic sunscreens.

With that being said, physical sunscreens remain popular for a variety of reasons. Since zinc oxide and titanium dioxide come from naturally occurring sources, they're often considered safer and/or more gentle on skin than chemical sunscreens. The "natural is better" messaging that's often communicated in contemporary advertising is powerful.

For some people, physical sunscreens really are the safer choice, though that's not because they're natural. It's simply because there are many, many more chemical UV filters than physical ones, and chemical sunscreens typically combine several filters for optimal stability and protection, so if a person has a reaction to a chemical sunscreen, it's easier and cheaper to swear off of the entire category than it is to undergo the arduous process of trial and error to determine exactly which chemical filter doesn't agree with their skin. Physical sunscreens are typically recommended for sensitive skin due to the lower risk of irritation or other reactions.

Chemical/Organic UV Filters

For people who don't need to stick to physical UV filters, chemical filters—also known as organic filters due to the carbon-hydrogen bonds they contain—offer an array of benefits. Chemical filters tend to result in far more cosmetically elegant products, with little to no white cast, lighter consistencies, and less chance of the heavy, greasy finish that often turns people off of sunscreen altogether.

Many chemical filters also offer greater UVA protection than physical filters, which is particularly important if you're using sunscreen in part to ward off early signs of aging.

So why doesn't everyone use chemical sunscreens?

Mainly, chemical sunscreens are often thought to be more irritating than physical filters. But while some filters, like oxybenzone, are known to be less suitable for sensitive skin, it isn't accurate to say that all chemical UV filters are inherently more irritating or sensitizing. Some may be more irritating to some people. Others might not. There are simply too many options in this category to generalize.

As of 2020, the United States FDA has approved the following ingredients as chemical UV filters: Aminobenzoic acid, **avobenzone**, cinoxate, dioxybenzone, **homosalate**, meradimate, **octocrylene**, **octinoxate**, **octisalate**, **oxybenzone**, padimate O, ensulizole, sulisobenzone, and trolamine salicylate.[11] The bolded ones are the ones you'll see most often on sunscreens here. And that's just the US. The US FDA is notoriously slow at approving new sunscreen ingredients, leading to a lag in innovation compared to other countries, particularly Japan and Korea. Once you start shopping for Asian sunscreens, you'll find even more, and many more advanced, chemical UV filter options.

Are Chemical Sunscreens Safe?

Over the last decade or so, proponents of the "natural is better" and "chemicals are bad" ways of life have mounted an effective campaign against chemical sunscreens, based on faulty interpretations of limited data.

Organizations like the lobbying group Environmental Working Group (EWG) claim that oxybenzone, homosalate, and octinoxate are "endocrine disruptors" that are hazardous to human health. Commercial media and independent bloggers have picked up these claims and spread them far and wide.

What's often lost among the fearmongering is the fact that the main study the EWG cites was conducted by feeding rats an enormous dose of oxybenzone over a short period of time.[12] A *Journal of the American Academy of Dermatology* study calculated that it would take 277 years of daily sunscreen application to replicate the systemic levels of oxybenzone in humans.[13] To date, no human studies have found any endocrine effect in humans, even though oxybenzone has been in use since the 1970s.

Part of this lag may be due to cultural differences. East Asian standards of beauty have historically favored very fair skin, and continue to do so even now. Very fair skin can be quite a feat to achieve and maintain when East Asian skin often tans easily in the sun. Preventing tanning and protecting fair complexions therefore demands an arsenal of sun protection products, ranging from umbrellas and visors to highly protective sunscreens suitable for everyday use. In the West, on the other hand, tan skin is often admired. Until relatively recently, sunscreen was considered an occasional use item—something you'd get when you were going to spend the day at the beach or park or on a hiking trail, rather than something you apply as part of your everyday routine.

It makes sense that East Asian brands would invest far more into researching and developing ever better and more cosmetically elegant UV filters than Western brands—the East Asian market, and the Asian market overall, demands them. For that reason, the price, performance, and protection (including the clearly stated UVA protection) of Japanese and Korean sunscreens makes them my go-to. That's why we'll focus primarily on Asian sunscreen types in this chapter.

Types of Sunscreens

As might be expected for a market as highly developed and competitive as the Asian sunscreen market, there are a huge variety of sunscreen types to choose from. Sunscreen is one of the most critical steps in a basic skincare routine, so take your time choosing one that meets your protection needs and looks and feels good enough to use every day. I've organized the basic types of sunscreens according to the skin types they generally work best for. As always, however, remember that exceptions exist to each rule. You may need some trial and error before you find The One.

Dry to Very Dry Skin

When looking for a sunscreen suitable for very dry to dry skin, there are a few common formulation tricks to keep in mind.

The most common ingredient you'll run into (and should avoid) is **alcohol denat**. Alcohol denat. has its place in cosmetics. It's a solvent, a penetration enhancer, and a quick and relatively reliable way to make a product dry down faster and more thoroughly, preventing the heavy, unpleasant residue that the product might otherwise leave behind. Unfortunately, alcohol denat. can also be drying, which is the last thing very dry or dry skin needs.

Also be on the lookout for **silica**. Sometimes used to create a matte finish or a slight blur effect in cosmetics, silica is a dessicant. Its drying effect sometimes extends beyond the product and into skin. In general, avoid silica if your skin is already dry.

Sun Creams

Cream-type sunscreens are often most suitable for very dry to dry skin. Generally, these contain a fairly high amount of emollient moisturizing ingredients, sometimes enough so that they can also replace the morning moisturizer step.

Normal Skin

As with moisturizers and other types of skincare products, normal skin is blessed to be able to use a variety of product consistencies, depending on what effect you're looking for. Normal skin can often get away with using more alcohol-heavy sunscreens, and a bit of silica might not hurt.

Sun Gels

Gel-type sunscreens (often called water gels) may be different than what you're expecting. These aren't the clear, goopy gels we often see on skincare and haircare shelves. An Asian gel-type sunscreen is simply a more watery and lightweight lotion with a slightly translucent appearance and a high humectant content. Gel sunscreens often contain alcohol to aid in their lightweight skinfeel. Their finishes can range from dewy to matte depending on the product and work well for normal skin. Alcohol-free gel sunscreens may also suit more dry complexions.

Oily Skin

In conversations with readers, I've found that those with oily skin are often the most reluctant to commit to daily sunscreen use, due to the perception that any sunscreen (especially one applied in the generous amounts required to achieve the full advertised protection on the label) will be suffocatingly greasy on their skin. Luckily, Asian sunscreens provide some great options for oily skin.

Sun Milks

Milk-type sunscreens often work extremely well for oily skin. These thin, liquid formulations generally give a very non-greasy finish and often contain silica and/or alcohol to promote a matte finish, effectively controlling the appearance of oil on skin. People often find that these also double as excellent mattifying face primers! Just watch out for those that contain a high amount of silicones, as they can produce a very shiny finish.

Other Sunscreen Formats

In addition to the main cream, gel, and milk-type sunscreens, several other formats exist. Stick sunscreens are a nice addition to use around the eyes, since the stiff, balm-type consistency of these doesn't run easily so will be less likely to sting the eyes. Powder, spray, and cushion sunscreens can serve as convenient ways to touch up sunscreen on the go. I don't recommend any of these sunscreens for primary use, however. It would be difficult to impossible to use them in the recommended amounts all over the face.

How to Apply (and When to Reapply) Sunscreen

Near the beginning of this chapter, we discussed the amount of sunscreen needed to achieve the full protection advertised on the product label: approximately ¼ tsp for your face alone, and an additional ¼ tsp or so for your neck and upper chest.

If you measure out any lotion with a measuring spoon, you'll see it's quite a lot of product. That's the main reason I don't recommend relying on the SPF in makeup or moisturizer for UV protection—it would be impossible to use that much of those products without looking absolutely ridiculous. That's also why the cosmetic elegance of your sunscreen is so important. Find a sunscreen that looks and feels good on your skin when applied in these very generous quantities.

Once you do, apply it generously every day, rain or shine, if you're going to leave the house. Most UV damage is not caused by the yearly trip to the beach, but by incidental sun exposure accumulating throughout the years. Your daily walk to the car or from the office to your regular lunch spot; your afternoon stroll with the dog. UVA in particular penetrates cloud cover. Maintaining daily protection is the best thing you can do for your skin.

It's often recommended to reapply sunscreen after two hours of sun exposure, due to the perception that UV filters (particularly chemical filters) destabilize and lose their effectiveness within that short time frame. Many sunscreens these days are photostable enough to remain effective even after two hours of sun exposure, but reapplication is still a good idea if you've sweated, gotten wet, or otherwise risked physically wiping off your sunscreen. Dab on more as thoroughly as you can, especially on high-exposure zones like cheekbones and the bridge of your nose.

And finally, once you've gotten a look at how much ¼ tsp is, don't worry too much about getting *exactly* the right amount on your face. Just be generous, apply approximately that much, and don't let fears of not doing it *perfectly* stop you from knowing that you're doing it *well*.

The SPF Conundrum

As a regulated metric controlled by government agencies worldwide, SPF seems safe, objective, and easily understood , right? Like many other aspects of skincare, it's not quite so simple.

Different countries require different testing protocols and standards for measuring SPFs, meaning that a sunscreen that qualifies as SPF 45 in one country may only earn an SPF 30 rating in another (or might exceed SPF 45, according to the second country's standards!). To further complicate matters, independent testing has exposed erroneously high SPF claims on products from major brands in major markets, including the US, the EU, Australia, and South Korea.

So how can we trust our sunscreens?

First of all, we remember that reaching a specific number is not our goal. Our skin doesn't have its own calculator to determine the SPF number on the product we use. Reaching a specific level of protection is. Yes, higher protection is always better—as long as the sunscreen we're using is cosmetically elegant enough for us to stand to use it in generous amounts every day.

Between an SPF 50 product that looks and feels like white greasepaint and an SPF 40 product that's lightweight and invisible, I will always consider the

SPF 40 preferable. I can use it daily in the correct amounts and receive the full protection, whereas with the cosmetically inelegant SPF 50 product, I'll likely end up skimping on it in an attempt to look normal or will end up rubbing a fair amount of it off in my desperation to blend away the white cast.

As you shop for sunscreens, look for reviews. I ignore sunscreen reviews that include any variation of the phrase "a little goes a long way," since, no, it doesn't. I pay attention to reviews from bloggers and influencers who I know to use sunscreen diligently and generously, and I particularly appreciate the ones who provide photos or videos of their application process. From there, I can check to see how well the products protected the reviewers. Any mention of burning, tanning, or freckling, and I know it's not the one for me.

It would be wonderful to be able to fully trust the SPF numbers on product labels, but as with all things born of capitalism, we can't. But we can compare reviewers' experiences with the claims brands make, and we can pay attention to how products fare on our skin. Personally, I simply look for a sunscreen that combines reasonably high SPF claims with notable cosmetic elegance. If my skin doesn't burn, tan, or freckle after use of the product, I consider it effective.

REFRAMING YOURSELF AS A PERSON WITH HEALTHY HABITS

"I know I should use sunscreen, but I can never remember to. I'm just not a sunscreen person."

"I do want to start a skincare routine, but I doubt I'd stick to it. It's just not my thing."

"I've been thinking about [exercising more, eating more healthily, going to therapy, insert anything you're pondering here], but I just can't commit to things like that."

Do any of these sound familiar?

Consciously and subconsciously, we all tell ourselves stories about ourselves every day: stories about the kind of person we are, the things we're capable of, and the things we aren't. Over time, for better or worse, those stories become our reality. Not because they're necessarily true, but because our belief in them has shaped our identity and made them true. Negative self-talk isn't always as clear-cut as "I'm trash and I'll never amount to anything special." Sometimes it's simply "I'm not the kind of person who can do [thing I know I should do]."

The first example can be just as damaging as the second, because these limiting beliefs about yourself hold you back from pursuing the changes that could help you feel better in your own life. There's a difference between being realistic about your limitations (for example, my 5'2" ass is never going to play for the WNBA) and kneecapping yourself with incorrect assumptions about your own potential.

Depression and anxiety can amplify these beliefs, but even if you don't suffer from either of these, you likely do indeed suffer. Just about everyone has limited themselves at some point because of their negative self-beliefs. Our perception of our own capabilities often shapes what we're able to accomplish and how much we're able to change our habits for the better. Therefore, practicing mindfulness of our own internal narrative can be a powerful first step in improving our lives. What we tell ourselves about ourselves becomes our identity, but identity isn't fixed. It's changeable, and we can consciously change it.

How?

In conversations with friends and readers, I often joke that it's all about brainwashing yourself. Specifically, brainwashing yourself into believing that you are actually the kind of person that you aspire to be yet currently believe you are not. "Brainwashing" is a strong word, but it isn't inaccurate.

I used to hate cleaning. Every apartment I lived in demonstrated that fact: dusty shelves, spotty mirrors, toilets overdue for a scrubbing. Even now, I don't particularly love the act of cleaning. It's not fun. But I do it every week, and I do it pretty thoroughly, because I stopped thinking of myself as a person who hates cleaning. Instead, I started thinking of myself as a person who loves relaxing in a clean and tidy space. That shift in identity transformed the weekly tedium of scrubbing and dusting from torture that I dreaded into a task that I welcome because I enjoy the results.

We can apply this kind of reframing to just about anything that we don't feel we're capable of. To go back to the example at the very beginning of this section, instead of thinking "I'm just not a sunscreen person," it would be more helpful to think "I'm a person who takes care of the health of my skin." Experiment with perceiving yourself differently and more positively. Once you've done it long enough, you'll wake up one day to find that you've made it true, and that you're better off because of it.

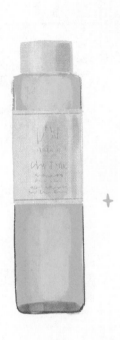

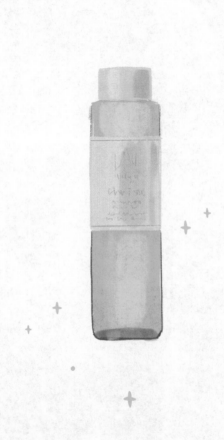

Chapter 5

TREATMENT: TARGETING ACTIVES FOR SPECIFIC SKIN CONCERNS

Congratulations! You've laid down a solid foundation of cleansing, moisturizing, and sunscreen, and you're ready to take on the complex but incredibly rewarding task of targeting and treating the specific skin issues that you'd like to change.

But first, a word of encouragement.

Spend enough time in skincare communities online or speaking with people in real life, and you'll hear some naysaying about skincare, particularly over-the-counter, nonprescription, mass market skincare. I've heard dermatologists say that no over-the-counter skincare is effective; I've heard estheticians say that no mass market skincare (that is, skincare you can purchase outside of their spas and clinics) is effective. I've heard both dermatologists and estheticians say that the only way to truly improve skin's texture and appearance is with treatments like peels, lasers, and injectable fillers. And I've heard plenty of people from all walks of life say that all skincare is a scam, that none of it works.

Sometimes these generalizations originate from a profit motive. Sometimes they originate in limited and often brand-provided product training, which is by its nature biased towards whatever brand is providing the training. Sometimes these generalizations come from simple ignorance of the research or from personal discouragement ("Nothing worked for me, therefore nothing works").

Luckily for those of us who either don't want to or can't afford to undergo cosmetic procedures or clinical treatments, these generalizations are wrong. Yes, ineffective and misleadingly marketed products exist. In fact, I'd guess that more skincare is ineffective and misleadingly marketed than not. But effectively formulated products also exist, and often at price points accessible to many of the people who can't spring for lasers, needles, or the knife. (For the record, I've never had any cosmetic procedures or treatments done to my face. I don't even get facials.)

Our task is to identify the products most likely to be effective for our particular skin concerns. With a little ingredient and formulation knowledge, that's not as daunting a task as it might first appear. We'll start with common categories of treatment products, then work our way into different skin concerns and the ingredients shown to benefit them most.

TYPES OF TREATMENT PRODUCTS

In beauty, especially Asian beauty, just about any product type can contain ingredients meant to address specific skin concerns. There are supposedly skin-firming face washes and acne-fighting lotions, spot-lightening toners and cell-protecting creams.

Just because the products claim special effects on their packaging, however, doesn't mean they live up to those claims. As we discussed in the moisturizer chapter, some product types simply don't lend themselves to effective formulations for targeted treatments and are unlikely to produce substantial results. Moisturizers belong to that category. So do cleansers. A product that's meant to be rinsed off your face immediately after application generally won't leave enough of its active ingredients behind (even if it contains an appropriate concentration of those active ingredients) to produce much of an effect on skin.

That may be disappointing to discover. It would be wonderfully convenient if we could kill two birds with one stone and address multiple skin concerns with a simple wash-and-moisturize routine. Plenty of products claim to do this. Someday they may actually live up to that claim. For now, removing cleansers and moisturizers from the list of products we use to treat skin issues still leaves us with a lot of options, and that's for the best. The more options we have, the greater the chances are that we'll find exactly what we need. All of the product types below may contain ingredients suitable for treating different skin problems.

I've listed these in the order in which they're usually layered in a Korean skincare routine, for two reasons. First, as you progress in your own skincare journey, you may find yourself using multiple types of products, and it will be easier to remember which order to put them in if you're used to seeing them presented that way. Secondly, the potency of these products as targeted treatments tends to increase from the thinnest type of product to the thickest—that's not a hard and fast rule by any means, but it is a useful rule of thumb to remember. So we'll start from the thinnest and usually weakest, and move up to the thickest and usually strongest.

Toners

Toners are thin liquid products sold in large volumes and intended for use immediately after cleansing. Broadly speaking, there are three types of toners, all with their own unique functions.

Toners almost always contain a very high amount of water as their base, a necessity to achieve the very runny consistency characteristic of this type of product. For that reason, beneficial ingredients that are most effective at very high concentrations won't do much in a toner. There's generally not enough room for an effective concentration of that type of ingredient. On the other hand, toners that use a water-based botanical extract as their base may provide some additional benefits. There are also some active ingredients that show significant effects at low concentrations, and those often appear in toners.

Astringent Toners

Applied by swiping over skin with a cotton pad or ball, astringent toners remove excess oil and dirt from skin after cleansing. Some also induce a temporary tightening effect. I'm personally not a fan of this category of product—in my opinion, if there's excess left to wipe off your face after you've already cleansed, then you need a better cleanser— but some people find them useful, particularly for very oily skin or in hot and humid climates. Astringent toners are generally characterized by **alcohol denat.** or **witch hazel** high in their ingredients lists.

Acid Toners

Acid toners also possess a cleansing function, though in a different (and, in my opinion, more beneficial way). An acid toner contains alpha hydroxy acids (AHAs) and/or beta hydroxy acids (BHAs), which are chemicals that help loosen and remove dead skin cells. Regular exfoliation with an acid toner can help to unclog pores and brighten and smooth the surface of skin. Further along in this chapter, we'll talk more about chemical exfoliants and what to look for in an acid product.

Hydrating Toners

Generally thicker than astringent or acid toners, hydrating toners contain a higher concentration of humectants to bind water to skin, delivering quick hydration to improve the texture and feel of dehydrated skin. These are the most common types of toners in Asian skincare. If a toner doesn't seem to be astringent or exfoliating, it's a hydrating toner. You may also be able to identify them by the prominence of hydrating ingredients like glycerin and hyaluronic acid in their ingredients lists.

Essences and First Essences

Moving a step up from toners, you'll find essences and first essences. Brands market these as having more targeted effects than toners, which primarily exist to cleanse or hydrate, so you'll see a larger variety of options in this category.

First Essences

First essences are a category of their own, and one that deserves special recognition.

The main ingredient of almost all first essences will be some form of yeast ferment extract, usually rice-based, typically the byproduct of sake or beer production. By breaking down compounds into smaller and theoretically more bioavailable pieces, fermentation is said to help ingredients better penetrate and benefit skin. First essences almost always claim skin tone brightening and anti-aging effects as their key features and are always intended for use immediately after cleansing. Their main ingredient is typically either **galactomyces ferment filtrate** or **saccharomyces ferment filtrate**, and they almost always have a thin, runny consistency, like toners.

Essences

Theoretically, an essence falls in between a toner and a serum in terms of concentration and potency. While most essences retain a primary hydrating or moisturizing component, they generally also claim some more targeted effect on skin, though less so than serums or ampoules. This "in-between" status can make essences feel less

134

effective and therefore less necessary than serums or ampoules, and in many cases, I'd agree.

The few essences that have impressed me have all had one thing in common: they've contained a high amount of an ingredient that benefits skin most when applied in generous quantities. Snail mucin, one of my longtime favorite skincare ingredients, fares better for me in essences than in serums, for example—its results for me seem improved when I'm able to slap it on thickly, rather than in the smaller amounts that smaller serum and ampoule packages dictate.

Serums and Ampoules

Although serums and ampoules are technically two distinct categories of products, I'm placing them in the same category here to make a point: in the vast majority of cases, brands use the terms interchangeably, making the distinction much more about marketing than it is about any particular formulation difference.

According to the marketing, a serum is a product formulated to target a specific skin issue and containing a potent concentration or combination of ingredients used to improve that skin issue. Serums typically come in smaller bottles than essences, further reinforcing the impression of higher concentration and potency. Ampoules, meanwhile, are said to be even more potent and concentrated than serums—they may come in single-use vials or other packaging form factors designed to encourage short-term usage with implied rapid results. In practice, however, there are 30ml bottles of product labeled as ampoules, and there are intensive four-week courses of products called serums.

The Marketing Factor

Don't get too hung up on different types of products, whether by limiting yourself to just one of each type or feeling that you need one of each type.

In the end, much of the differentiation between essences, serums, and ampoules is marketing. While serums and ampoules allegedly contain higher dosages of beneficial ingredients, the results prove it isn't always the case. Sometimes the serums and ampoules are simply thickened to give the appearance of a more concentrated product, suggesting greater potency (and enabling the brand to justify charging a higher price per ounce). And certain ingredients simply don't need to be present in particularly high concentrations (or would be too irritating or damaging to use in high concentrations). As you'll see in the ingredients section below, for example, chemical exfoliants work especially well in toners.

Now that we've covered the basic types of treatment products, the real fun begins: identifying the ingredients best suited to your needs!

SUPERSTAR SKINCARE INGREDIENTS AND HOW TO FIND THEM

Skincare ingredients research has a long way to go. Academically credible, peer-reviewed, large-scale, long-term studies take time and money. There is far less time and money available than there are potentially beneficial ingredients to study, especially at the rate that brands push out exciting-sounding new products featuring tantalizingly named new ingredients. Competition drives innovation, and the highly competitive Asian cosmetics market tends to reward brands that push the envelope with esoteric plant extracts and flashy formulations.

There's a place in my heart (and my skincare closet) for both the narrow minority of extensively researched ingredients and the vast universe of newer and less tested ones. In this chapter, we'll focus primarily on the former category, since those are the ones that we turn to for the treatment of primary skin conditions. Many of these ingredients affect skin in multiple ways, so at the end of this section, you'll find a chart to further help you narrow the field to the ones most suited to your needs.

Primary Actives

I consider an ingredient an "active" when it is capable of substantially affecting the actual structure or function of skin, rather than simply temporarily altering its moisture levels or surface texture. Primary actives are the most potent in this category. When delivered in effective formulations and used consistently for extended periods of time, primary actives can purge out deep clogs, accelerate and optimize skin cell turnover, stimulate increased collagen production, and more.

With great potency comes great responsibility, however. Primary actives must be used with caution, since they all carry the potential for some undesirable side effects. In addition, they must be formulated effectively to achieve their primary objectives. Luckily, enough research exists on these ingredients for us to know how to identify a good formulation.

Alpha Hydroxy Acids (AHAs)

Suitable for: Fine lines, rough skin texture, hyperpigmentation, and some types of acne.

What it does: Alpha hydroxy acids work primarily by breaking down the bonds that hold dead skin cells together, allowing the dead cells to slough off faster and more evenly than they would otherwise. With proper use and sun protection, this smooths skin texture and fades hyperpigmentation over time.[14] AHAs can also help clear whiteheads and closed comedones by uncovering deep clogs and allowing them to purge out. Since AHAs are water soluble, they act on the outer surface of skin and will not penetrate sebum.

Secondary benefits: Alpha hydroxy acids are humectant and therefore sometimes recommended over BHAs for dry skin.

What to look for and what to watch out for: The three main AHAs you'll see in skincare are, in order of strength, **glycolic acid**, **lactic acid**, and **mandelic acid**. If you prefer a product you can use fairly regularly, look for an AHA concentration of 5–8%. If you'd rather use a stronger product less frequently, consider peel-strength AHAs, which generally contain 15% or more of the active ingredient. Additionally, AHAs work best at a low pH. An AHA product with a pH between 3 and 4 is ideal.

AHAs are photosensitizing: they render skin more sensitive to sun damage. For this reason, you must use sunscreen properly and consistently when using any AHAs to exfoliate your skin. The photosensitivity persists for 7 days after the last application of an AHA product, too. I know you're not going to just stop using sunscreen for no particular reason, but it's especially important when dealing with photosensitizing actives.

What kinds of products to look for: To maximize effectiveness, AHAs should be applied on bare or close to bare skin, so lower concentration, regular use AHAs work well in toners. Peel-strength AHAs most commonly come in serum form.

What kinds of products to avoid: Cleansers that contain AHAs are unlikely to provide much, if any, of the exfoliating effects expected of an AHA.

Ascorbic Acid (Vitamin C)

Suitable for: Fine lines, loss of elasticity, and hyperpigmentation.

What it does: L-ascorbic acid (L-AA) vitamin C fades dark spots and hyperpigmentation by inhibiting melanin production, and its strong antioxidant activity can also help prevent existing melanin from darkening due to oxidation. Additionally, L-AA stimulates increased collagen production.[15] Consistent use for extended periods of time can result in firmer, smoother skin.[16]

Secondary benefits: Since L-AA is a potent antioxidant, regular use can protect skin against free radical damage caused by UV exposure, pollution, stress, and other external factors. While this protection won't replace your primary protection of a properly applied sunscreen,

it is an excellent supplement to SPF and general safe
sun practices.

What to look for and what to watch out for:
Unfortunately, L-AA is notoriously unstable and prone
to oxidation. For best results and the longest shelf life,
it should be formulated in a product that also contains
tocopherol (vitamin E) and ferulic acid, at a pH between
3 and 4. Concentrations of 15% and above produce the
quickest and most visible effects on skin. The combination
of an acidic pH and a high concentration can make an
L-AA serum irritating for some people, however.

L-AA products should not contain added dyes, which may
conceal product darkening due to oxidation, which reduces
the effectiveness of the product. A vitamin C serum should
be clear or champagne-colored when first opened, and I
advocate tossing it when it is darker than yellow. Keep
L-AA products in the refrigerator after opening to extend
shelf life a bit.

What kinds of products to look for: Since L-AA
oxidizes and loses effectiveness quickly, look for serums
sold in small bottles that can be used up within a month or
so. Around 20–30 ml is ideal. Opaque airless pump bottles
are optimal for extending the product's shelf life, though

dark or opaque dropper bottles are acceptable as well. L-AA in a clear bottle is likely to be a waste of money, since constant exposure to light will hasten the product's demise.

What kinds of products to avoid: Even if effectively formulated, toners and creams that contain L-AA will tend to lose potency before you can use them up, making them a waste of money and product. Additionally, while shelf-stable vitamin C derivatives like **magnesium ascorbyl phosphate (MAP)** and **sodium ascorbyl phosphate (SAP)** do solve the oxidation issue, less research currently exists to support brightening and collagen-building claims in products that utilize these derivatives.

Azelaic Acid

Suitable for: Rosacea, redness, acne, clogged pores, and hyperpigmentation.

What it does: Originally developed as a topical acne treatment due to its antibacterial and exfoliating properties,[17] azelaic acid has gained popularity as a treatment for hyperpigmentation as well. Thought to directly eliminate abnormal melanocytes, which are responsible for hyperpigmentation disorders like melasma and for post-inflammatory hyperpigmentation from acne, azelaic acid can selectively fade abnormal pigmentation without affecting normal skin tone.[18]

Secondary benefits: Azelaic acid's anti-inflammatory properties make it a promising active for reducing redness overall, and some people report a reduction in the appearance of their pores after consistent use.

What to look for and what to watch out for:
Most of the successful studies of azelaic acid to treat acne, hyperpigmentation, or rosacea have used it at concentrations of 15–20%, which at the time of this book's publication are considered prescription-strength. Over the counter (OTC) azelaic acid products offer lower concentrations so require a longer period of use before seeing results.

Azelaic acid is a milder exfoliant than AHAs and BHAs, making it more suitable for people with a low tolerance for chemical exfoliation, but it may still cause irritation and dryness, especially in those with sensitive skin.

What kinds of products to look for: Azelaic acid is available in cream, gel, and serum formulations, all of which can be effective. Concentration is more important than format for this ingredient, so choose the type of product most usable for your skin.

What kinds of products to avoid: Like other actives, azelaic acid is unlikely to be comparably effective in wash-off products like cleansers.

Beta Hydroxy Acids (BHA)

Suitable for: Clogged pores, blackheads, and acne-prone skin.[19]

What it does: Like alpha hydroxy acids, beta hydroxy acids are chemical exfoliants that break down the bonds holding dead cells to the surface of skin. Unlike AHAs, BHAs are oil soluble, so they can penetrate into open pores, where they can loosen sebum clogs. Their oil solubility also makes BHAs particularly suitable to oily skin.

Secondary benefits: BHAs are also anti-inflammatory, a secondary benefit for acne-prone skin.

What to look for and what to watch out for: In the West, **salicylic acid** is the most commonly used BHA, while Asian brands often opt for the milder **betaine salicylate**. A daily use BHA should contain around 2% salicylic acid or 4% betaine salicylate, concentrations at which most people find the products effective without being too irritating. Stronger BHAs do exist for occasional use. BHAs are not as pH-dependent as AHAs, though a lower pH will still boost their performance (while slightly increasing the risk of irritation).

BHAs can be drying, so if your skin is on the dry side, avoid applying all over face. Use only on the areas that need it—typically the T-zone.

What kinds of products to look for: Similar to AHAs and vitamin C, BHAs tend to work best when applied to clean skin. Toners and pre-moistened wipes (like the acne pads many of us remember from our teenage years) deliver the active ingredient well.

What kinds of products to avoid: Outside of toners and acne pads, BHAs most often appear in cleansing products. Since cleansing products are rinsed off immediately after application, they're unlikely to provide benefits comparable to leave-on options. If you do want to try a BHA cleanser as an addition to your routine, look for one that contains an effective percentage of the active ingredient and that includes instructions to leave the cleanser on for a minute or two before rinsing. This will give the BHA more time to penetrate and produce the advertised effects.

How to Layer Actives

You may have noticed that I've described three different actives as working best when applied to bare skin, and you may be confused about how to go about layering multiple actives in one routine if more than one of them should go on bare skin.

As long as each of the actives products is fairly thin and light, without emollient or occlusive residue, layering two or three after cleansing shouldn't reduce the effectiveness of each active. Just wait a few minutes in between each layer to allow it to penetrate and dry down, then move on to the next. Consider your actives an extra step in your cleansing process. That will make subsequent product additions less confusing, too.

Topical Retinoids (Vitamin A)

Suitable for: Fine lines, wrinkles, loss of elasticity, hyperpigmentation, and some types of acne.

What it does: Retinoids are a class of exceptionally beneficial skincare ingredients. Derived from vitamin A, retinoids alter gene expression in the skin, essentially reprogramming it to turn over faster and more healthily. Photodamaged skin sheds and is replaced by more rapidly grown new skin. Some retinoids also reduce collagen breakdown, stimulate increased collagen production, and counteract the natural thinning of skin with age[20].

Secondary benefits: Retinoids are also antioxidant and may help protect skin cells from free radical damage.

What to look for and what to watch out for: Retinoids come in both prescription and over-the-counter forms. Tretinoin and retinol are two of the most commonly seen ones for aging skin concerns.

Tretinoin, or retinoic acid, is the most extensively research-supported retinoid. It's only available by prescription in the US and is so potent that even concentrations as low as 0.005% produce significant effects. As of the publication of this book, the maximum concentration of tretinoin that I've seen is 0.14%.

While tretinoin's potency is a major draw, its potential side effects are major drawbacks. Tretinoin users often experience significant dryness, irritation, flaking, and peeling, especially near the beginning of treatment before skin has adjusted to the medication. To minimize these side effects, start with a low dose of tretinoin, work up slowly to daily use, wait at least twenty minutes after cleansing before applying, and consider buffering it by applying over other products rather than on bare skin.

Although observed to be much less potent than tretinoin—twenty times less potent, according to some researchers—**retinol**, an OTC retinoid, carries a far lower risk of side effects like redness, irritation, dryness, and peeling. Like tretinoin, retinol can help thicken the epidermis and encourage collagen production, resulting in reduced fine lines and wrinkles and improved elasticity. According to current research, concentrations of around 1% retinol are effective.

Retinol is much weaker than tretinoin, however, with some researchers observing that it's "twenty times less potent" than its prescription cousin. Retinol must be converted by skin into retinoic acid in order to work. The conversion breaks down the retinol; the final result is a concentration of retinoic acid that's a fraction of the original concentration of retinol.

As you browse retinol products, you'll likely stumble across some whose active ingredient isn't actually retinol, but rather some retinol derivative, like **retinyl acetate**, **retinyl palmitate**, or a number of other ingredients with "retin" somewhere in the name. Although marketed as comparably effective retinol alternatives, retinol derivatives are far less extensively researched and generally less potent than retinol. That isn't always a bad thing, however. While retinol generally causes less irritation than tretinoin, many people do still experience the typical retinoid side effects when using an OTC retinol product. Retinyl palmitate in particular is a gentler way to ease skin into retinoids.

Due to their mechanism of action, which accelerates the growth of new skin and the shedding of old skin, retinoids, like AHAs, are photosensitizing. Use a high-protection sunscreen generously and consistently with them.

What kinds of products to look for: Retinoids can function well in a variety of product formats, including serums and creams. In fact, creams with an effective concentration of retinoids are often a less irritating choice, especially if applied over other products. Keep in mind that retinoids do degrade with light exposure. Dark, opaque, and/or airless packaging is best.

What kinds of products to avoid: I suggest avoiding retinoids that don't disclose the exact concentration of their active ingredient. It implies that the brand is aware they aren't including an effective amount and are simply using the retinoid as a claims ingredient. The product may be perfectly nice in other ways, but it shouldn't be considered a primary retinoid product.

Using Primary Actives Safely

Now seems as good a time as any to clarify that just because you *can* use all the actives above (in the sense that no one is stopping you from procuring them all) doesn't mean you *should*.

As we discussed, all the actives above come with potential drawbacks. AHAs and retinoids are photosensitizing (again, liable to give you some redness and inflammation). BHAs and azelaic acid can be drying. L-AA vitamin C serums can be irritating. (The one I like the most stings when I apply it.) Additionally, overuse of AHAs and/or BHAs leads to overexfoliation and dehydrated skin, while even moderate use of a strong retinoid can cause short-term flaking, peeling, and general dryness and sensitivity. Oh, and don't forget—using multiple actives can cause side effects to pile on top of each other. The sensitivity caused by retinoids or overexfoliation will make the vitamin C even more irritating, for example. (If you're wondering if you can ever win this battle, don't worry, you can.)

It is possible to use multiple actives at a time. I do it. That doesn't mean that it is advisable for everyone—some people's skin handles tons of actives perfectly fine, while others can't take it. If you're new to actives, it's best to err on the side of caution and assume your skin might not be able to take it.

As with all other new skincare products, only introduce one new active at a time. I normally advise people to give a new product at least a week or two to see how well their skin tolerates it, but in the case of actives, I suggest giving each new active a month before adding anything else to your routine, since some side effects, like overexfoliation, take time to appear.

Finally, remember that real results take time. You should feel an improvement to your skin texture fairly quickly with AHAs and BHAs, since their effects manifest on the upper layers of skin, but vitamin C and retinoids, which affect the growth of skin and collagen, typically need several months of consistent use to produce visible results. Just because you don't see any change after a few weeks doesn't mean the product doesn't work. Patience is key with skincare, as with so much else in life!

Secondary Actives

Like primary actives, secondary actives are well researched and capable of altering the structure and function of skin. Unlike primary actives, however, secondary actives don't drastically alter skin's turnover rate or require especially acidic pH formulations, making them a generally gentler option with less risk of side effects.

As with any other cosmetic ingredient, however, secondary actives can cause reactions if your skin happens to be sensitive to these ingredients. Continue to introduce products one at a time in order to gauge whether your skin agrees with them before fully committing.

Ceramides

Suitable for: Dry skin, dermatitis, compromised skin barrier due to overcleansing and/or overexfoliation, premature fine lines, and loss of elasticity due to dehydrated skin.

What it does: We discussed ceramides briefly in our section on moisturizers, but they deserve an extra mention in this section due to their importance to a healthy skin barrier. Your skin produces ceramides naturally, and these waxy lipids are crucial to helping skin hold moisture in and keep contaminants and irritants out. This makes them crucial to repairing a damaged moisture barrier or strengthening one that has grown weak due to age.

Secondary benefits: Ceramides are excellent occlusive ingredients, so can work well to moisturize skin even in a healthy state.

What to look for and what to watch out for: For optimal penetration and barrier repair, ceramides should be combined with cholesterol and fatty acids or sphingosines. There is some debate about the optimal ratio of ceramides, cholesterol, and fatty acids, but since the vast majority of cosmetics will not list the exact percentages of each ingredient for you to calculate their ratios anyway, your best bet is to look for products whose ingredients lists at least contain ceramides, cholesterol, and either some oils or sphingosines, such as phytosphingosine or oligosphingosine.

What kinds of products to look for: Due to the fatty nature of this ingredient and its support ingredients, ceramides tend to perform best in lotions and creams. They can be found (and can work well) in lighter products as well, but those will generally provide less moisture overall.

What kinds of products to avoid: If you're layering multiple products in a K-beauty-style skincare routine, avoid using ceramide-heavy products early in your routine. They can slow absorption of your subsequent skincare layers, making your routine take longer and potentially decreasing the effectiveness of the products.

Copper Peptides

Suitable for: Fine lines and wrinkles, loss of elasticity, photodamage, and hyperpigmentation.

What it does: The peptide GHK, listed in cosmetics ingredients as tripeptide-1, naturally occurs in human plasma (and other bodily fluids). So where does this active get this fascinating name? Well, GHK has a "strong affinity for copper," combining with copper in human tissue to form GHK-Cu.[21]

Like so many other beneficial substances, its presence in our bodies decreases as we age. Luckily for our skin, topically applied GHK-Cu has been shown to stimulate collagen production in aging skin. This may be due to the fact that GHK is a collagen fragment, so its presence in skin may fool skin into producing more collagen as a response to presumed collagen breakdown.[22] Theoretically, this will result in firmer and less wrinkled skin over time. Research also suggests that GHK-Cu may improve wound healing and therefore skin regeneration, which is good news for those concerned with sun damage and the visible aging process.[23]

Secondary benefits: GHK-Cu is also antioxidant and anti-inflammatory.

What to look for and what to watch out for: GHK-Cu penetrates skin better when encapsulated in a lipophilic delivery system (basically combined with a lipid/fat), as it is when listed as Matrixyl® 3000, which combines the peptide with a palmitic acid. I have had success with copper peptides even without the lipophilic encapsulation, however, so I wouldn't consider that a must. Look for a stated concentration of 1% or above, and look for copper in the ingredients list as well as tripeptide-1.

At lower pH levels, copper will separate from the GHK. For this reason, it's often stated that copper peptides cannot be used in the same routine as acids. As long as you wait a few minutes in between your acidic products and your copper peptide products, however, you should be fine.

What kinds of products to look for: Serum and cream products are your best bet with GHK-Cu, although a toner-type product with a stated concentration of 1% or above may work well too.

What kinds of products to avoid: Wash-off products like cleansers and single-use or occasional-use products like masks are unlikely to be effective.

What Are Peptides?

As you browse for your next skincare purchase, you may notice a strong emphasis on peptides, particularly in the anti-aging categories. They're impressive-sounding ingredients, and brands capitalize on that to market their products.

In junior high (or high school; my memory is fuzzy), we learned that amino acids are the building blocks of proteins. Peptides are simply chains of amino acids. You can figure out how many amino acids a given peptide ingredient contains by its prefix: dipeptides contain two amino acids, tripeptides contain three, and so on.

Not all peptides offer the same benefits to skin, and not all have been studied extensively enough to support their use in cosmetics, at least as competitors to better-established actives like retinoids. Your best bet when you see an enticing peptide product is to research the specific peptides it contains in order to get an idea of what results you might expect.

Niacinamide (Vitamin B3)

Suitable for: Hyperpigmentation, blotchiness, sallowness, fine lines and wrinkles, loss of elasticity, and compromised barrier function.

What it does: As you might have guessed from the long list above, niacinamide is one of the true heroes of skincare—a secondary active capable of targeting a wide variety of common skin issues. Best known for its ability to effectively fade hyperpigmentation without the unpleasant side effects and photosensitivity of primary actives like retinoids and AHAs, niacinamide also improves your skin's elasticity, can reduce the appearance of fine lines and wrinkles, and improves sallowness in aging skin.[24] It also stimulates increased ceramide synthesis, leading to a stronger skin barrier, and has anti-inflammatory benefits as well.[25] What's not to love?

Secondary benefits: Niacinamide is an antioxidant and may help protect against free radical-induced cell and DNA damage.

What to look for and what to watch out for: Niacinamide shows up in a huge variety of products these days, and I never find its presence in an ingredients list problematic. For a dedicated niacinamide product that you expect to achieve some of the effects mentioned above, however, I would look for a product that contains it at a concentration of at least 5%, which the previously referenced studies have shown to be effective. It may still be helpful at lower concentrations, especially when formulated with other supplementary ingredients that target the same concerns, but only at 5% or above would I consider a product a "niacinamide product," no matter what form it comes in. Niacinamide is especially effective when combined with N-acetylglucosamine.[26]

What kinds of products to look for: You'll typically find 5% niacinamide in serum-type products, although I see no problem with a cream, toner, essence, or any other product that contains an equal amount of this ingredient.

What kinds of products to avoid: Niacinamide in cleansers or other wash-off or single-use products won't have much, if any, effect on your skin—this is an ingredient that needs to be used consistently over time in order to see results.

* * *

At this point, you may be feeling overwhelmed, especially if you're interested in the effects of more than one primary or secondary active. To help you find the best ingredients for your concerns, use the information in this chapter. And don't worry about having to add a new product to your routine for every active you'd like to incorporate: many products use more than one in a single formulation. Niacinamide and retinoids often appear together, for example; niacinamide and ceramides do, too. Instead of looking for one product for each active, figure out which actives you'd like to try and see if you can find products that combine some of them.

FINDING JOY IN THE THINGS WE LEARN ALONG THE WAY

The lists of ingredients I give in each section of this book are by no means comprehensive. If I were to include every single skincare ingredient out there, with research and evidence of its beneficial effects, this book would be an encyclopedia, and it would go out of date quickly— new ingredients are being researched and marketed all the time, especially in the faster-paced East Asian cosmetics industries.

I wanted to keep the focus on ingredients I've personally used and seen success with. My attitude towards giving product reviews and skincare advice has always been descriptive, not prescriptive: Skin is so individual that I can only tell you what has worked (and hasn't worked) for me, not what will (and won't) work for you. The personal discovery and trial and error elements of skincare are unavoidable. And that, as I hope you'll see, is not a bad thing at all.

What I want to do is provide you with a starting point for your journey. While no one can promise you that any particular ingredient or product will do for you what it has done for them, I am focusing on ingredients whose effects are supported by research and that I and many others have found effective for our skin. They're tried and true, and many of them were my starting point as well.

From here, where you go is entirely up to you. As you browse products marketed for your skin concerns, pay close attention to their ingredients. Look up the ones that are most heavily featured or that sound the most intriguing to you. Find out what research has been done on them and what others have to say about them. With skincare as a self-care tool, the learning can be as important as the doing.

In fact, learning about skincare has done as much to improve my general mental health as actually using the skincare has. Growth is powerful, especially in the battle against depression.

If you've gone through an extended depressive episode, I imagine you know what I mean. Hour by hour and day by day, we're tempted to give in to the gloom. To stay in bed a little longer (or to get back in bed the instant things feel overwhelming). To put off that chore or project for one more day. To find reasons to stagnate, because the alternative feels too taxing for our limited energetic and emotional resources. Depression is *heavy*. In the moment, we're often tricked into believing that the solution is to sit down, figuratively. To put down the burden, to rest.

In that state of rest, however, the hours and days and weeks and months slip away. We stagnate. But as we stagnate, a part of ourselves recognizes this and raises the alarm. Life is short, and the part of ourselves with dreams and goals (or at least a desire for stability and comfort) cries out that we're wasting time, letting our lives slip away.

Out of the conflict between the part of us that just wants to rest and the part of us that wants to move forward comes guilt. The guilt is often a response to a lack of growth, a cessation of forward movement.

Entirely by accident, I found that both learning about skincare and applying it were effective and pleasurable ways to short circuit that guilt. When we learn—actively seeking out new information, integrating it with our existing knowledge base, and finding ways to put it into practice—we grow. When we grow, we feel more in control of our existence. That sense of control, of empowerment, is potent, and it can positively affect our motivation in other areas of our lives as well, gradually helping us build a ladder to climb out of the depths of depressive episodes.

Skincare served as a uniquely ideal vehicle for me. It wasn't my job (at the time), so I didn't feel any external pressure to do it in a certain way or at a certain pace. It interested me, so I derived pleasure in simply learning for the sake of learning. And, of course, what I learned had practical benefits, as I grew more confident in choosing products and saw real improvements in my skin. All of this combined to make my hobby rewarding and intrinsically motivating. Ultimately, that's what made it stick and what changed my life.

As you begin choosing your first actives and finding products to try, take a moment to appreciate what you've learned so far and to look forward to what you will learn as you go. You don't need to know everything all at once. No one is grading you, no one is judging you, and no one expects you to achieve expert status with your first serum pick. Skincare is something you're exploring for you and you alone. You deserve the chance to pursue it for your own enjoyment. Out of that pursuit will come natural growth, all of which you've earned.

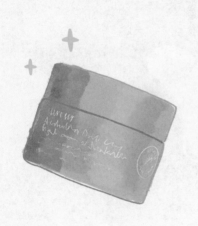

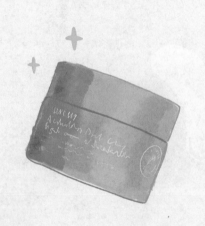

Chapter 6

REFINEMENT: PERFECTING THE SURFACE OF YOUR SKIN

In the previous chapter, we discussed actives, which are shown to produce substantial changes to the structure and function of your skin. So what comes next?

If you've structured your routine by the hierarchy of skincare needs of sustenance, protection, and treatment—in other words, cleansing, moisturizing, sunscreen-ing, and treating specific skin issues—you're solid. If each step in this routine works well for your skin, you're already well on your way to dramatically improved skin that will retain its health and appearance for far longer than it would have otherwise.

Not everyone enjoys the act of researching and experimenting with skincare enough to proceed beyond the basic routine. If you don't see yourself deriving joy from delving even deeper into the skincare world, you can stop there and still feel confident that you've done your skin (and your habits) a great favor.

If you do find yourself curious to learn more, or if you'd like to see just how much more you can improve your skin, then read on. This chapter is about the "refinement" level of the hierarchy of skincare needs. Here, we'll discuss how we can build upon the basics to achieve something much closer to perfection—the absolute best your skin can look at this moment in time and for as long as you continue.

You can find refining ingredients in every category of skincare we've already covered, but there are some additional product types especially suited to this stage of your skincare journey. We'll discuss those additional product types first, then cover some of my favorite ingredients for complexion refinement.

FACE MASKS: NOT JUST FOR SPECIAL OCCASIONS

You've come a long way already, and at this point, you may have a clear idea of what your skincare routine will look like. You might even have picked up a few new products. But we haven't even gotten to the really fun part!

For most people, face masks are an occasional indulgence: a boost before a big event, or an added treat in your regular nighttime skincare routine to transform it from a daily task into a relaxing spa night. If chosen wisely and used consistently, however, they can be so much more than that. The ones that work best for you can also be incorporated on a regular basis if you're willing to go that far (as I am). Having a couple of masks on hand also helps spice up your regular routine with some variety, staving off tedium and giving you something to look forward to.

Clay Masks

Arguably the most recognizable mask type for Western audiences, clay or mud masks can be a useful occasional treatment for oily or congestion-prone skin. They can be made with a variety of different types of clay, each with unique mineral content and claimed benefits; some of the more common ones you'll see are bentonite, kaolin, Dead Sea, Aztec, and French green clay.

Clay masks are generally marketed as "clarifying" due to their ability to absorb oil[27]: they can temporarily reduce the amount and appearance of oil on the surface of your skin and draw sebum out of open pores, making them look cleaner and smaller. They are also sometimes marketed as having a tightening or firming effect, although it's likely that these effects are due to the hardening clay and your skin tightening as it dries rather than any actual change in your skin.

Overuse of clay masks can dry out skin and lead to sensitivity and irritation, so exercise restraint when using them, and choose a clay mask appropriate for your skin type. Clay masks these days don't all harden to a dry, cracked crust while sucking all the moisture out of your skin. Many brands now make creamier clay masks that contain emollient moisturizing ingredients. These will have less raw oil-absorbing power but also suit dry or sensitive skin better.

To use, apply to clean skin, then wait for as long as the package instructions specify before rinsing off. Due to their drying tendencies, I like to use clay masks on nights when I can follow them up with a sheet mask or a hydrating or moisturizing wash-off mask.

How Often Can I Use Each Type of Mask?

Everyone's skin is different, but in making mask recommendations to readers, I have a few basic rules of thumb about frequency of mask use. These are generalizations, so consider your skin's own needs and the instructions provided with your masks as well.

Clay masks shouldn't be used more than once a week due to their drying properties. For normal skin like mine, once every two weeks works well. People with dry or sensitive skin should use them even less frequently.

Exfoliating scrubs shouldn't be used more than once a week, unless they're made with exceptionally gentle exfoliating particles, like konjac or rice, which can be used more frequently.

Sheet masks can be used daily—as I certainly do. In fact, if you have the time, budget, and inclination, you can enjoy them twice a day. I've done so at various points in my life, and I'm not the only one.

Nourishing masks can be used a few times a week if desired. The only reason I don't support daily use

of these is because the act of rinsing them off may
begin to cause symptoms of overcleansing.

Exfoliating Scrubs

Scrubs are another category that you'll probably recognize
even if you're unfamiliar with Asian skincare products.
These products use a physically abrasive element to
slough off dead skin cells when you massage them on,
leaving softer, smoother skin behind—some popular scrub
types are sugar, salt, and ground-up apricot shells. Many
also contain moisturizing ingredients to further nourish
your skin during use.

I like exfoliating scrubs once in a while, especially to get
a perfectly smooth canvas under makeup, but most scrubs
should not be used too frequently. Just like chemical
exfoliants, exfoliating scrubs can damage skin's moisture
barrier with overuse, leading to irritation, sensitivity, and
dehydrated skin. For this reason, I also prefer gentler
exfoliating particles. Konjac or rice grains are the softest,
while sugar scrubs can be more or less abrasive depending
on how much sugar the scrub contains. I stay away from
salt scrubs for face, since salt grains are sharper-edged

and more likely to irritate. I never use scrubs that contain ground-up apricot pits or walnut shells, since those are also too sharp and abrasive for most facial skin. (Although they are nice on body skin, which is tougher and can take more exfoliation!)

To use, massage them gently onto your skin, then rinse off. Some exfoliating scrubs are also marketed as wash-off masks with additional skincare benefits. If the instructions indicate to wait a certain amount of time before rinsing, feel free to do so as well.

Sheet Masks

Sheet masks are my personal favorite refining product by far. I use one at least a few times a week and sometimes go through phases where I use them nightly. When I do, I always see a marked improvement in the overall appearance of my skin.

Consisting of a large volume of hydrating or moisturizing essence soaked into a cotton, silk, or cellulose pulp sheet that's cut to fit over the face, sheet masks use the physical occlusion of the sheet to increase the liquid's penetration into skin. This enables skin to take in far more product than it otherwise could, since the sheet helps prevent the liquid from evaporating and keeps skin in a moist and more permeable state.[28]

Sheet mask essences generally contain a large proportion of water and humectants, making their main benefit the intensive hydration they deliver to skin. Most also contain ingredients marketed to provide additional effects, like brightening, calming, or firming. While I wouldn't rely on a sheet mask to achieve long-term effects, since the concentrations of the additional ingredients tend to be quite low, the short-term hydration itself is worth the extra effort for me. The diversity of featured ingredients and claimed results also makes sheet masks a low-risk way to play around with ingredients I find interesting but am not ready to incorporate into my routine in the form of a daily use product just yet.

When choosing a sheet mask, there are a few precautions to keep in mind. The extended period of time the mask stays on your skin, as well as the large volume of essence, mean that the effects of any irritating ingredients can be amplified. If you suspect a sensitivity to any particular ingredients, avoid those in sheet masks. As a general rule, I also avoid sheet masks that contain alcohol or fragrance, since those are common irritants.

Instructions vary by sheet mask, but in general, I find sheet masks perform best when used after any hydrating products and before moisturizers, and I like to leave them on longer than the package directions specify—my ideal sheet mask wear time is about forty-five minutes. Do not rinse unless the directions specify otherwise, and make sure to seal in the hydration with a moisturizer afterwards!

Nourishing Masks

Nourishing masks are a diverse category. No matter what your skin type or skin troubles are, you'll likely find something in this category marketed towards you. There are hydrating gel masks, moisturizing cream masks, firming masks, oil balancing masks, warming masks to increase circulation, cooling masks to soothe irritation, and everything in between. What these all have in common are their directions: you apply them to your face, wait for however long the instructions suggest, then rinse off.

Of the types of masks I've discussed in this section, I personally use wash-off masks the least—I can count on two fingers the number of wash-off masks that I consider worth the extra labor of putting them on then rinsing them off. You may feel differently.

The main advantage of nourishing masks is that the selection of these is comparable to the selection of sheet masks available on the market. No matter what ingredients you're interested in trying or what effects you hope to achieve, it's likely you'll be able to find a nourishing mask to fit your desires. Like sheet masks, they're a fun way to experiment with intriguing ingredients, without committing to a daily use product.

Spa Night: Combining Multiple Masks in a Single Routine

When I was a teenager, my best friend and I spent many weekend evenings doing "spa night." We'd pull out whatever face masks and mask samples we had lying around and bond by giving each other amateur facials and trading tips we'd picked up from the magazines we devoured every month.

I still love bonding with friends over skincare, and I still love doing spa nights. These days, though, there's more method to my madness.

If you want to use several different mask types in one session, here's my preferred order for doing them, and why:

First: Exfoliating scrubs or peels. Remove dead skin first to clear the way for any clarifying, hydrating, or nourishing masks to achieve maximum results.

Second: Clay masks. Sweeping away the debris from the upper layers of your skin gives clay masks better access to your pores, allowing them to pull out more sebum and general gunk than they could otherwise.

Third: Hydrating masks. Exfoliating and clarifying masks work to remove impurities from your skin but can also remove moisture. Using a hydrating mask after a purifying mask takes advantage of the increased permeability of your skin to replace what's lost with fresh hydration and nutrition.

Fourth: Moisturizing masks. Masks that deliver emollient moisture to skin should go after those that deliver water and humectants. The emollients will help seal in the hydration for maximum retention.

Do note that I'm not saying every spa night requires all four mask types. Do just one with your regular routine, do two, do three, or do all four—it's up to you. But if you do more than one, follow the order provided for best results.

Now that we've covered some of the additional ways you can enjoy skin-refining ingredients, it's time to get down to business: the ingredients themselves!

REFINING INGREDIENTS AND WHAT THEY DO

We've gone beyond the basics now and into the part of skincare that I find really *fun*—folk remedies, herbal medicine, and botanical extracts. Cleansers, moisturizers, sunscreens, and heavily researched actives are the meat and potatoes of a skincare routine. Refining ingredients and product categories are the seasonings and the desserts. They're perhaps less scientifically proven, but they can make or break the experience. They can also enhance the products and your routine in powerful ways. I consider some of these ingredients as indispensable to my face as retinoids and sunscreen.

But What About the Science?

There is less scientific research behind the ingredients discussed in this chapter, and indeed behind most popular cosmetic ingredients today. Not every cosmetic ingredient comes with an extensive pedigree of academic and/or clinical research, for a very simple reason: money.

In vivo (conducted on living humans) testing is difficult and expensive, especially compared to *in vitro* (conducted on cells in a petri dish) testing. Large-scale, long-term, double-blind, placebo-controlled studies are especially difficult and expensive. There simply isn't enough interest in, say, the cosmetic effects of the topical application of some random Korean mushroom to justify the outlay of research funds that could go to other, more pressing topics. Where research into cosmetic ingredients does exist, it's often funded and/or conducted by cosmetics brands themselves, so an element of bias creeps in.

With all that being said, I obviously don't view these less "proven" ingredients to be less worthy. An absence of rigorous testing doesn't necessarily equate an absence of real benefits to skin.

I eat healthily (more or less), exercise, and go to the doctor when I'm ill, but I also experiment with herbal supplements and other practices to further optimize my health. Similarly, I cleanse, moisturize, and use actives and sunscreen, but I also experiment with less proven ingredients like the ones in this chapter to further optimize my skin.

Approach these ingredients and others like them with an open mind. You may discover holy grails for your skin that no academic journal could have predicted. Just be aware that since less research exists on them, there are no established standards for concentration in a given product. As a reminder, the higher up in the ingredients list they appear, the more the product will contain.

Centella Asiatica (Pennywort, Gotu Kola, Tiger Grass) Extract

Suitable for: Redness, irritation, sensitivity, sunburn, and acne inflammation.

What it does: The anti-inflammatory and wound healing properties of centella asiatica extract[29] and centella asiatica derivatives make them a good fit for skincare marketed to calm redness and swelling, like the kind you might experience from an active acne flare-up or that sunburn that you're totally never going to experience because you use sunscreen diligently now. I've had some positive experiences with centella products and especially like them when I've overexfoliated or had a misadventure with a new product.

Secondary benefits: There are claims that centella asiatica's wound healing potential makes it useful for consumers interested in delaying or reducing the visible signs of skin aging.

What to look for and what to watch out for: Many Korean products categorize centella asiatica products as "Cica," so searching for this term when you browse for products will bring up plenty of possibilities. When you read ingredients lists, also keep an eye out for madecassoside, asiaticoside, madecassic acid, and asiatic acid. These are the main active compounds in centella asiatica. They're often isolated and used as standalone ingredients, and they carry the same potential benefits as centella asiatica extract itself.

What kind of products to look for: I've had success with centella products in all the main categories, so I suggest starting by looking for whatever type of product you have room in your routine for, whether that's a toner, serum, cream, or even sheet mask. Centella is an especially nice addition to sunscreens, since it can help cut down on inflammation caused by sun exposure.

What kind of products to avoid: None. Even a centella cleanser has worked out well for me, since centella can offer some immediate relief from sensitivity and irritation.

Honey and Propolis

Suitable for: Dryness, dehydrated skin, rough texture, irritation, sensitivity, and some forms of acne.

What it does: Honey is not just a delicious condiment or pet name for a loved one. It's also one of my most-loved skincare ingredients. Its humectant and emollient compounds help to smooth and moisturize skin without leaving an oily finish. Honey may also assist in wound healing,[30] and its antioxidant content could provide protection at the skin barrier from free radical damage.[31]

I've often found honey-based products noticeably calming for irritated skin.

While less moisturizing than honey, propolis offers its own array of benefits. The most relevant for skincare purposes are its antimicrobial and anti-inflammatory properties, which can help prevent and calm breakouts without inflicting more irritation on skin the way many common acne-fighting actives do.

Secondary benefits: Honey and propolis both have fairly significant antioxidant content.

What to look for and what to watch out for: Bee sting allergies are common, so if you are allergic to bee stings, it's best to play it safe and either avoid honey- and propolis-containing products or patch test them extensively before adding them to your regular skincare routine. As for what to look for, honey and propolis seem to perform best when used in high concentrations in cosmetic products, so look for products that list these ingredients high on the ingredients lists.

What kind of products to look for: To maximize its potential as a moisturizing ingredient, seek out moisturizers and richer serum products containing honey. Propolis also works nicely in moisturizers, but in my experience delivers the most notable benefits in lighter products applied closer to skin, like toners, essences, and serums. Honey and propolis also enhance face masks of all kinds, though I favor honey in nourishing masks and propolis in sheet masks.

What kind of products to avoid: In my experience, no particular product types suffer from the addition of honey or propolis, although honey may make products that need to be lightweight, like sunscreens, heavier than they would otherwise be.

Glycyrrhiza Glabra (Licorice Root) Extract

Suitable for: Dark spots, hyperpigmentation, dullness, redness, and irritation.

What it does: It may taste nasty to some (including me), but licorice has a storied history as a medicinal herb, with references to its use found in ancient documents from Egypt, India, China, and the Greek and Roman empires. Today, you'll find it in a variety of skincare products. Licorice is comparatively well researched, even for the treatment of skin conditions like atopic dermatitis,[32]

against which its anti-inflammatory effects have been shown effective. In cosmetics, licorice root often appears in spot-fading and skin-brightening formulations, since it can inhibit melanin production.[33] It's one of my favorite ingredients for evening out my skin tone, since it fades both excess pigmentation and blotchy redness.

Secondary benefits: Some components of licorice root extract also show strong antioxidant activity.[34]

What to look for and what to watch out for: Licorice root pairs well with other brightening ingredients and actives, particularly niacinamide, so look for it in products that contain both. Don't worry too much about the concentration of licorice root extract. Even in studies done for the treatment of atopic dermatitis, licorice root extract appears effective at concentrations as low as one to two percent, so there's little need to look for it at the top of an ingredients list.

Glycyrrhiza glabra is the most commonly used type of licorice you'll see in a cosmetic product, but some brands use glycyrrhiza uralensis instead.

What kind of products to look for: While licorice root extract can enhance just about any product, I have found the best results with watery products like toners and first essences, as well as with sheet masks. Its anti-inflammatory properties also make it a soothing addition to products that otherwise have increased potential for irritation, like exfoliating acids.

What kind of products to avoid: None.

Panax Ginseng Extracts

Suitable for: Fine lines, wrinkles, loss of elasticity, dullness, dark spots, and hyperpigmentation.

What it does: Ginseng has a storied history in traditional Chinese and Korean herbal medicine: it's commonly used to promote general health and vitality, to boost immunity, and to improve resilience against environmental stressors. In skincare, it may boost collagen production,[35] resulting in smoother and firmer skin with fewer visible signs of aging. There's also evidence that it can suppress the production of melanin to help reduce and prevent dark spots and hyperpigmentation.[36] Many of my absolute favorite skincare products contain ginseng and ginseng-derived ingredients—I've personally experienced dramatic improvements to my skin texture, tone, and elasticity when using ginseng.

Secondary benefits: Like many of the other ingredients in this list, ginseng is anti-inflammatory. It also shows potent antioxidant ability.[37]

What to look for and what to watch out for: The most commonly used part of the ginseng plant is the root, and you may see a couple of different types of ginseng root extracts on product labels. While both "white" and "red" ginseng root extracts come from the same plant, white ginseng root extract involves first drying the root, then putting it through the extraction process. The costlier and presumably more potent red ginseng root extract, on the other hand, comes from ginseng roots that are steamed and dried before extraction. The steaming step releases additional beneficial compounds, called ginsenosides.

Ginsenosides are also sometimes included in products as free-standing ingredients. Some products also incorporate the extracts of ginseng berries and other parts of the plant. Those may provide additional benefits but are unlikely to provide equivalent benefits as the root extracts.

What kind of products to look for: I have personally found ginseng products most effective when they come in a serum or cream.

What kind of products to avoid: The primary benefits of ginseng require consistent use, so ginseng in a cleanser is unlikely to do your skin much good, since you rinse it off right away.

Snail Mucin/Snail Secretion Filtrate

Suitable for: Fine lines, wrinkles, dehydrated skin, rough texture, irritation, sensitivity, sunburn, and some kinds of acne.

What it does: The better question is, what does it *not* do?

As you might have guessed from the fact that my blog is named *Fifty Shades of Snail*, I love snail in skincare. I've loved it since my first hesitant uses of my very first snail product, and that love has never faded. In fact, it's only strengthened over the years and with experience and an ever-growing range of ingredients to compare snail to.

Snail mucin, sometimes labeled as snail secretion filtrate, is exactly what it sounds like: snail slime, filtered and purified.

Unlike many of the other ingredients in this list, the use of snail mucin for healing purposes did not originate in Asia.

Ancient Greek texts reference it as a treatment for burns and other wounds, and it apparently saw a revival as both topical and ingested remedy in eighteenth and nineteenth century Europe.[38] These days, however, it's emblematic of the Korean skincare trend of the early to mid 2010s, its use in cosmetics representing a perfect blend of appreciation for natural ingredients, advancement of cosmetic research, and willingness to try very strange-sounding things on one's face.

In addition to humectant and emollient components that make snail mucin an excellent non-greasy hydrating and texture-smoothing moisturizer, snail mucin demonstrates wound healing properties[39] in some studies. Other studies (and my personal experience and that of many of my readers) suggest it may help repair sun-damaged skin and reverse some signs of photoaging,[40] as well as reduce atrophic (indented) scarring,[41] which commonly appears after acne or chicken pox.

The collagen, elastin, and amino acids in the snail mucin also help form a flexible protective layer over your skin, increasing its protection against both water loss and external irritants—I find snail especially helpful when I've damaged my moisture barrier through overcleansing or overexfoliation. Finally, its antimicrobial components may help ward off acne. That, combined with its healing potential, make it another excellent supplementary ingredient in an acne-fighting routine.

Secondary benefits: Snail mucin has some antioxidant and anti-inflammatory properties.

What to look for and what to watch out for: Like honey and propolis, snail mucin seems to perform best when incorporated into products in high concentrations. I prefer snail products that actually use the snail slime as the base of the product—in other words, snail at the top of the ingredients list, denoting that it is present in greater concentration than any other ingredient in the formula. My longtime favorite snail-based products are more than ninety percent snail secretion filtrate. I generally pass on snail products that contain less than sixty percent snail mucin, since I've found them markedly less effective at the things snail mucin excels at.

There is some crossover between dust mite and snail allergies,[42] so if you have a dust mite allergy, exercise caution when trying out snail products. Don't despair, though. I have a mild dust mite allergy and use snail mucin products without issues.

What kind of products to look for: In the high concentrations that I recommend, snail mucin gives products a thick (though non-oily) and distinctively stretchy consistency. This makes it most suited to thicker essences, serums, and moisturizing creams.

What kind of products to avoid: The same consistency that makes snail work so well in thicker moisturizing products also makes it less suitable for watery products like toners.

How is Snail Mucin Extracted?

Discomfort around the idea of snail mucin in skincare sometimes comes from unfamiliarity with how it's acquired.

The process varies by supplier, but in general, snail farms feed the snails a carefully controlled diet and allow them to roam on some mesh or net surface. Their slime is collected from there. Some suppliers may stimulate the snails to produce more slime by manually stimulating their shells. Others use mild electrical shocks to stress the snails, a method with which I am not comfortable. The most humane but likely least economical method is simply to let the snails move around and produce slime naturally, without external stimulation or stress. All of my favorite snail products are made by a brand that sources its snail mucin from a supplier that uses this method.

Most brands don't advertise how their suppliers get their slime, but it doesn't hurt to ask, and there's usually some way to get in touch with the brand via social media or from their websites. And it may be reassuring to know that snails are not killed to extract their slime. Constantly replacing snails that can continue producing slime as long as they live would be pointlessly costly.

Seaweed/Sea Kelp/Algae Extracts

Suitable for: Dry or dehydrated skin, rough skin texture, hyperpigmentation, and loss of elasticity.

What it does: Last in this list but not last in my heart, seaweed, sea kelp, and algae extracts are more than just delicious additions to soup and nutritious wrappings for sushi rolls. Rich in beneficial bioactive compounds, the extracts of these marine plants are outstanding refining ingredients for skin. At the most basic level, their humectant and emollient properties work well for hydrating skin and holding moisture in; they work unusually well for firming and smoothing texture, resulting in a more naturally youthful appearance. They also show promise for inhibiting melanin production, thus helping reduce and prevent dark spots and hyperpigmentation, and may slow the breakdown of collagen and elastin in skin, delaying signs of aging.[43]

Secondary benefits: Seaweed, sea kelp, and algae extracts contain high amounts of antioxidants, which protect against free radical and UV-induced skin damage.

What to look for and what to watch out for: Cosmetics ingredient suppliers work with numerous species of seaweed. Some of the most common you'll see in beauty products are *laminaria digitata, laminaria japonica, corallina officinalis, ecklonia cava, hizikia fusiformis,* and *undaria pinnatifida,* though you may also see seaweed, sea kelp, and algae listed on their own, without a species specification. Fermentation increases the bioavailability of the beneficial compounds in seaweed, so fermented seaweed extract, sometimes listed as sea kelp bioferment, is ideal. Seaweed seems to do the most good when included in high concentrations, so keep an eye out for it in the top half of a product's ingredients list.

What kind of products to look for: These ingredients provide the most benefit when used in moisturizing, leave-on products, so look for them in essences, serums, and moisturizers. They also perform well in face masks.

What kind of products to avoid: None. Pile it on with abandon if you find seaweed agrees with your skin!

On Extracts and Expectations

As we discuss specific ingredients and what they can do for your skin, it's important to remember that an ingredient is not a promise. This holds true even when the ingredient is a lab-produced active, manufactured in a consistent manner to consistent standards and identical across all producers. It's even more true when it comes to botanical extracts and many other naturally derived ingredients.

A lot of variables come into play when working with natural ingredients. The nutrient composition of the plants themselves depends on factors like growing region, season, soil quality, and farming methods.

Sea kelp extracts provide a visible demonstration of this: high-quality ones will vary in color depending on when they were harvested. Harvesting and extraction methods can also affect the final result. Extracts aren't standardized for potency or purity. One ingredient supplier's camellia sinensis extract may be much more concentrated and high-quality than another's, for example, although both extracts would appear under the same name in an ingredients list. And your skin's individual quirks are the greatest variable of all. As we often say in the skincare community, YMMV—your mileage may vary.

Seek out products that contain the ingredients you're interested in trying or already know work well for you, but manage your expectations. Reading reviews of the products you're eyeing can help give you a better idea of their potential for your skin. So can gaining an understanding of which ingredients certain brands excel in. Some brands specialize in certain ingredients and either grow and extract their own or provide transparency into where they source their ingredients. Both bode well for their extract quality.

Keep an open mind as you experiment, but remember—an ingredient is not a promise. Instead, it's a sign of potential.

SKINCARE TOOLS

In recent years, the variety of skincare tools and devices available to regular consumers has grown dramatically. It's not just cleansing aids and facial rollers, either. Home versions now exist for microneedling, a treatment formerly only administered by professionals, and that's just the start.

I'm covering skincare tools in this chapter rather than the Treatment chapter because in my opinion, none of these devices are fundamental to an effective skincare routine. Some may indeed give skin a moderate boost, so can be helpful as additional means of refinement. Others, however, are downright dangerous.

Cleansing Tools

Meant to be used with your facial cleanser, cleansing tools are typically marketed as providing either a deeper cleanse than hands alone, or as adding exfoliation to your regular cleansing routine, or both.

Konjac Sponges

Made from the root of the tuberous konjac plant, konjac sponges are small and springy, with a texture just rough enough to gently slough off loose, flaky dead skin cells without exfoliating too harshly for daily use. As a bonus, squishing a dab of cleanser in a wet konjac sponge will foam it up more effectively than lathering the same product between your palms, which can make gentle, low-foam cleansers more satisfying to use.

Electric Cleansing Brushes

You know how electric toothbrushes promise to clean teeth more thoroughly by oscillating much more rapidly and frequently than hand brushing can achieve? Electric cleansing brushes offer the same experience, except for your face. Like higher-end electric toothbrushes, some electric cleansing brushes also incorporate sonic technology to further loosen debris caught in hard-to-clean spots, like within your pores.

Is washing your face with the skincare equivalent of a vibrating electric toothbrush a good idea? That's highly dependent on your skin's tolerance to manual stimulation and exfoliation, as well as on the brush head you choose. If you're removing makeup and sunscreen before cleansing as needed, and using effective cleansing products, it's unlikely that your skin needs a deeper cleanse than what you'd achieve by washing with your hands instead of a cleansing brush. Using an electric cleansing brush every day also increases your chance of overexfoliation. If you want to try one of these tools, choose the softest brush head available, consider only using it once a day, and cut back or discontinue any other exfoliation until you see how well your skin tolerates the device.

Facial Massage Tools

If you're drawn to the aesthetic of indulgence—spa facials, heady scents, relaxing with a bottle of wine in a candlelit bubble bath after a long day at work—then facial massage tools may appeal to you.

198

Proponents of facial massage claim that by increasing circulation to the skin, it stimulates collagen production, resulting in firmer, more youthful-looking skin over time. However, as chemistry PhD and beauty educator Michelle Wong has pointed out on Instagram, just because massaging skin increases circulation and increased circulation can stimulate collagen production, that doesn't mean that massaging skin *will* stimulate collagen production.[44] There's little evidence that the act of facial massage, rather than whatever products are being massaged into skin, affects skin's structure or function.

On the other hand, gentle facial massage can have some positive short-term effects. It can help reduce puffiness from water retention and may relax facial muscles, especially if you're prone to frowning or otherwise tensing your face involuntarily.

If you do decide to get a facial massage tool and become confounded by the selection of different stones from which they can be made, or worry that the inexpensive models are inferior to the outrageously priced ones, don't be. No matter which type of fancy rock the tools are made from, they'll all perform the same function, so just choose the one that resonates best with you aesthetically (or spiritually) so that you'll enjoy using it more. As for price, costlier facial rollers *may* be better constructed and more durable than the inexpensive ones. Or they may simply be the exact same product produced by the exact same factory, packaged more nicely and marked up to the heavens.

If you suffer from acne, use massage tools with extreme caution or not at all. Massaging active pimples can push bacteria deeper in and further out from the original site of infection, worsening the breakouts.

Gua Sha Tools

Practiced in traditional Chinese medicine, *gua sha* therapy involves a practitioner forcefully scraping a smooth stone implement—the *gua sha* tool—across the client's skin in long strokes, with the direction of their strokes based on traditional theories of the energy channels in the body. Skin is typically lubricated with an oil first, but even so, the strokes are meant to be strong enough to bruise. Long stripes of dark red or purple bruising will crisscross a client's back by the end of the treatment.

Gua sha practitioners can also treat the face (without the vibrant bruising), but thanks to online video tutorials, many skincare enthusiasts now do it to themselves at home. As long as you've used enough facial oil or cream underneath to prevent friction irritation, and as long as you use a fairly light touch, you won't cause yourself harm. On rare occasions, I use a *gua sha* tool under my eyes to minimize puffiness in that area. Generally, however, I consider it too much work for too little reward to do on a regular basis.

Facial Rollers

Most often made from pretty stones like green jade, purple jade, or rose quartz, facial rollers consist of a polished stone roller on a small handle. To use, roll it in long strokes on skin. These are particularly popular for use over facial serums or sheet masks, with fans claiming the rollers help product absorb more fully into skin.

Like *gua sha* tools, these can help reduce puffiness by encouraging lymphatic drainage in the face. Chilled facial rollers also feel nice on overheated or inflamed skin. Don't apply too much pressure when you use them, and don't expect spectacular long-term results, but enjoy the relaxation!

Home Microneedling Tools

Out of all the device categories here, this is the only one that I feel confident in advising everyone to avoid like the plague.

Microneedling is a well-researched treatment to stimulate increased collagen production in skin. In a clinical environment, skin is punctured repeatedly with sterile microneedles, inducing "a wound healing cascade": the controlled trauma of the needle punctures initiates the body's wound healing process, ultimately leading to the growth of more new collagen and elastin in skin.[45] It's most often used cosmetically to address skin sagging, wrinkles, scars, and stretch marks. Needle length varies, with longer needles used to stimulate collagen production and shorter ones used to enhance the penetration of topical products.

Regular, properly spaced out microneedling sessions performed by a dermatologist or qualified aesthetician and followed up with appropriate aftercare are known to work. That's not the question. The question is whether untrained laypeople should be attempting to do this at home, at their own discretion. The answer, in my opinion, is a resounding "NO!"

As mentioned above, microneedling involves repeatedly wounding skin by puncturing it with needles. The tools used in dermatologists' offices and reputable medspas are sterilized to medical standards. A soak in rubbing alcohol at home is not the same thing. And as you can imagine, poking hundreds or thousands of tiny holes in your skin carries a significant risk of infection. On top of that, improper technique or damaged or poorly constructed home microneedling tools can cause permanent scarring. Finally, professionals can work with you to determine the optimal frequency of your treatments. Microneedling isn't a one-and-done procedure. Repeated visits are necessary to see results. Doing it too often is counterproductive, and not doing it enough won't help, either.

Whether you're considering a dermaroller or a dermapen, the two most popular amateur microneedling options on the market, just don't do it.

Exploring Skincare Devices

Cleansing, massage, and amateur microneedling tools are just the tip of the iceberg of the skincare devices on the market today. New technology and new gimmicks emerge at a regular pace (and on a schedule that likely correlates strongly with the schedule of major industry trade shows every year). I haven't even touched on microcurrent and LED light therapy devices in this book. I've never found either trend compelling, even with the science backing them up, because of the relative expense of the devices and my own laziness about using anything beyond topical products at home. By the time this book is published, there will likely be even newer and more hyped skincare accessories for me to ignore.

You aren't me, and you may be more willing to commit money and labor to a home skincare device. And that's great. As with refining cosmetic ingredients, I support everyone exploring what interests them and seeing where their interests lead, as long as they're making your selections in a relatively methodical manner. While some devices, like konjac sponges and facial rollers, are inexpensive and pose relatively little risk to the health of your skin, others are much more costly and/or significantly more hazardous to skin when used incorrectly.

At the consumer level, most information about new skincare technologies trickles down from the brands to the major beauty and women's websites and magazines, as well as to some independent content creators on social media. The information you'll hear about the devices at this level will probably be overwhelmingly positive, at least at first. That's the nature of marketing, and to some degree, pretty much all content created with the cooperation of a brand or vendor is marketing. So look beyond the gushing features on Refinery 29 and the regurgitated press releases and brand photography on social media.

If you feel confident in your ability to read scientific papers, search for the technology on Google Scholar. Once you locate some research into the technology being used, pay attention to how the studies were conducted. The closer they are to the conditions in which an end user would experience it, the better. *In vivo* studies are always superior to *in vitro*. Once you've checked out the research, you should have a better idea of what you can expect (and what you can't) from the device.

If you don't feel confident in your ability to read scientific papers, seek out content creators who are. Within the skincare and beauty communities, you'll find some influencers with serious scientific backgrounds. They generally make their credentials clear, understand how to interpret data, and work to explain the science behind skincare products and devices in terms that laypeople can better understand. When you're unsure whether to trust a brand's claims about their innovative new products, content creators like these can help.

Most of all, if you do decide to try some promising skincare device, remember: real progress takes time! As you do with your skincare products, give devices a few weeks or months to show results. Use them consistently as directed and take regular progress photos along the way. Giving them a chance to work is the best way to find the ones that do work for you.

TAKE THINGS ONE STEP AT A TIME

At this point, you likely have a clearer idea of what you'd like to include in your skincare routine; you may even have begun to get products and start using them already. Everyone who now has an established routine has been there, and many of us felt the same way once we started seeing all the possibilities: a mix of excitement and confusion, heads swimming with both visions of improved skin and questions about how the hell to get there.

If you're feeling overwhelmed, take a step back and take a deep breath. The most important thing to remember now is that you'll get the best results by taking everything one step at a time.

When I started exploring skincare and K-beauty back in the first half of the 2010s, I and others like me had very little guidance. There were a few blogs started by the very early adopters of the Korean skincare trend, of varying helpfulness. The best of them—many written by women who have since become close friends of mine— provided critical information on the basics of skincare (the importance of cleanser pH, the function of well-established actives and secondary actives) and delved as deeply as they could into what research existed on the unfamiliar and sometimes bizarre new ingredients they encountered. Others took a less scientific stance but provided honest and clear product reviews. Still others served mostly as unofficial mouthpieces for the brands beginning to see the value in the international beauty market. Even those blogs contributed to our collective knowledge base, though. Their reworded press releases and brand-provided product photos allowed the international audience to find out about new releases.

The thing is, everyone back then—from iconic bloggers like Kerry Thompson of *Skin and Tonics* and Cat Cactus of *Snow White and the Asian Pear*, all the way to the newest of the newbies asking their first tentative questions in the Asian Beauty community on Reddit—came at it from an equal position. We all wanted to try everything, and we did, with abandon.

Snail mucin essences. Creams containing ground-up starfish. Cleansers with the texture of lightly smashed marshmallows, packaged in heavy glass jars. If it existed, was available on one of the Korean export sites, and was weird enough to catch our eyes, we bought it, we tried it, and we shared our thoughts about it. The collective spending on products that we had little to no information on was through the roof, especially since the high shipping costs and long shipping times of the K-beauty vendors of the time encouraged infrequent but large hauls. Hundreds of dollars at a time for boxes full of products that failed to work out for our skin more often than not. We bought packs of foil samples and hoarded the free samples that came with our purchases.

It was chaos. Necessary chaos that built a foundation of English-language ingredient, product, and brand information from the ground up, but chaos nonetheless, especially for our faces. I'm fairly certain that everyone in the community at the time experienced at least one terrible breakout or facial rash after wildly testing something new. There was a widespread and in some cases truly devastating mass breakout due to a preservative failure and microbial contamination incident involving a popular product (which didn't even contain anything unfamiliar to Western consumers—its featured ingredients were aloe and propolis!). Much fun was had, but at the expense of many wallets and sometimes faces.

Not to sound too old and self-righteous, but we did all that so that eventually others wouldn't have to. Especially so that people who just wanted to find better solutions for their skin, rather than engage in skincare as a hobby and creative outlet, could just find better solutions for their skin. Which leads me back to you.

One step at a time is key. As I've mentioned before, it's best to add only one new product to your routine at a time, giving the new product at least a week or two (preferably more) so that you can at least make sure nothing in it disagrees with your skin. One step at a time goes beyond that, though. It also means only adding the steps you find your skin truly needs, rather than adding every step some brand or beauty vendor tells you your skin needs.

This is especially crucial in discussions about Korean skincare. If you're familiar at all with the K-beauty trend, you've most likely heard all about the mythical "Ten Step Korean Skincare Routine," which seemingly every beauty journalist has covered at one point or another in the past half decade or so. And the more you hear about this Ten Step Korean Skincare Routine, the more it can seem necessary. I've fielded probably hundreds of questions from readers asking for recommendations to fill certain slots in the routine, and learned after some probing that they're not even sure what to expect from adding another product—they just think they need to. They've taken the concept of the Ten Step Korean Skincare Routine as a template that must be completed.

It is not. Being a completist is beneficial in many areas of life, from home improvement projects to open-world video games filled with Easter eggs, but it is not always beneficial and not always necessary in skincare. Instead of thinking of the Ten Step Korean Skincare Routine as a template, think of it as a rough guideline for what order to use products in, or even simply a general list of possible product categories to buy. Because the fact of the matter is, the Ten Step Korean Skincare Routine is a marketing creation. Not an instruction manual. Which takes us to a very important topic to cover when we're talking about cosmetics and beauty capitalism: the sometimes dirty tricks that brands and marketers employ to convince us to purchase their products.

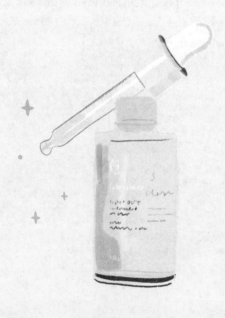

Chapter 7

THE UGLY SIDE OF BEAUTY

When I made the choice to tie skincare to self-care, I knew I would be walking a very fine line. The pursuit of beauty is often—and rightly—perceived as hazardous to one's self esteem and mental health.

The distinction comes, I think, from who we allow to set our expectations, something that applies to more than just beauty and skincare. Take fitness, for example. Most people would benefit both physically and mentally from more exercise. Striving to improve our personal fitness levels as much as we can within the constraints of our schedules, budgets, and any physical limitations is generally a rewarding endeavor. When the standard we're working to meet is simply our own personal best or even just "better than before," we can celebrate our progress at whatever pace we experience it, no matter how "small" our achievements may appear compared to others'. We can enjoy our growth more, stick with our efforts more consistently, and cope more readily with any setbacks we encounter.

On the other hand, when we attempt to meet a standard set by others, to achieve an ideal that has nothing to do with our own bodies and life circumstances—to try to reshape our bodies in the image of professional fitness instructors or models, for example—we often find ourselves disappointed in our own failure to live up to that external goal. A feeling of futility makes it easier to give up. We lose sight of the real gains we've made to our health due to frustration at not making the imagined gains we've set ourselves up to expect.

Everyone is different. Everyone grows at a different pace and in unique ways. But that's not always the message we hear when we look for external guidance and motivation. It's even worse when those external inspirations, those depictions of the ideal bodies that we're promised if we just follow the program and work hard enough, aren't real in the first place. Unfortunately, this scenario is all too real and all too common. Fitness programs are often sold using images of bodies that are either surgically altered or digitally edited. Perfection is already an unhealthy goal to set for one's body; it's an even more toxic goal when the depictions of perfection aren't even real.

The same goes for skincare. So many brands advertise their lotions and potions using photos of models who have been expertly made up, lit, photographed, and then digitally edited into absolute flawlessness. Not a wrinkle or a pore to be seen, much less any other more minor irregularities of tone or texture. Depending on your region and the shamelessness of specific advertisers, the message may be implicit or explicit, but the message is always the same: our products will give you this complexion, and this complexion is what you need to be beautiful.

That message wouldn't be as toxic as it is if not for the fact that just about every culture throughout history tells stories that equate physical beauty with personal worth, and just about every culture throughout history tells stories that establish physical beauty as a prerequisite to acceptance, love, and happiness. From childhood onwards, we're taught to admire beauty not just for its aesthetic appeal, but because beauty is cultural shorthand (and often seen as a shortcut) to other qualities we desire, from intelligence and virtue, to breeding and success.

All of this primes us, as adolescents and adults, to acquire the products we believe will help us achieve it, and to fear the consequences of failing to possess beauty.

Brands *know* this. This set of assumptions—the superior value of beauty and the necessity of beauty for love and happiness—underlies the vast majority of beauty marketing. That makes decoupling external beauty from internal worth a necessary task, both for beauty content creators like me and for beauty content consumers like you.

When I was younger, I consumed beauty media and products from a place of fear. I feared being unattractive by society's standards because I feared missing out on all the things that society says belong to the beautiful. These fears made me susceptible to all sorts of scummy advertising tactics.

I bought makeup that didn't suit me because it was shown on the lovely face of a lovely model arm in arm with a lovely, adoring boyfriend. I scrubbed my face raw with products sold via deceptive before-and-after photos depicting a "regular" girl's transformation from a scowling sufferer of full-face acne into the radiantly beaming owner of a perfectly spot-free face. I saved up and spent hundreds on creams endorsed by glossy magazines, never realizing that (a) those endorsements were likely purchased, and (b) the creams contained nothing special to justify their eye-watering prices. All the while, I was miserable. I obsessed over every "blemish" and couldn't understand why all my best efforts hadn't given me inhumanly perfect skin, and I was convinced that no one would ever want me and no one would ever love me if I couldn't discover the secret to that inhumanly perfect skin.

It was irrational, but it's all too common. My guess is that it may be even worse today, now that amateur photo editing apps allow everyone with a smartphone to airbrush their own pores and "imperfections" into oblivion.

I'm older now. I clearly still enjoy consuming beauty media and beauty products. The difference now is that it doesn't come from a place of fear, but from a place of enjoyment and self-love. The fact that I still value conventional standards of beauty enough to actively pursue them remains problematic, but I no longer believe that a freckle or pore or even a pimple (the horror!) will impact anything about my life whatsoever. I value beauty enough to enjoy feeling pretty, but not enough to fear that losing it will affect anything but my own face. Instead, I enjoy skincare and beauty on their own merits, because to do something I enjoy is an act of care for myself. That's where I hope to take you.

One of the first and most crucial steps in that journey is to recognize the ways in which advertising works to create and exploit insecurities in their target audiences. They're very good at it. That means we must be very good at arming ourselves against it.

Let's go back to imagery in advertising.

Brands don't photograph their spokesmodels simply to show off their beautiful skin. Those gorgeously shot ad campaigns tell narratives that teach you how their products are supposed to make you feel. Luxury brands dress classically beautiful actresses in high-end fashions, adorn them with expensive beauty, and feature them in images dripping with wealth and elegance. Youth-oriented brands depict fresh-faced young models and pop stars frolicking through flower-filled meadows or at the center of attention at the club. These are aspirational narratives that tell you how you'll feel and who you can become if you buy the products. They're selling a dream more than a face cream. And the advertisement of this dream tells you anything of substance about the content of the products themselves.

It doesn't always get better when the ads are transparent about what's in their products, unfortunately. There are a number of ways to make a mediocre product sound outstanding. After reading the earlier chapters of this book, you may already be able to spot these tactics more readily than before.

COMMON SKINCARE MARKETING TACTICS AND WHY THEY'RE MISLEADING

In my ideal world, every skincare advertisement would include the product's complete list of ingredients, and every skincare consumer would have the basic ingredient literacy needed to understand them. We do not live in my ideal world, however, as evidenced by the fact that I currently own zero cats instead of a dozen. Brands are perfectly aware of most consumers' lack of ingredient knowledge, and they capitalize on that shamelessly. The use of claims ingredients and intimidation marketing are two of the most often-deployed ways they do so.

Claims Ingredients

As the name might imply, claims ingredients are included just so the company can make certain statements about the product.

Cosmetics labeling and advertising is regulated by the FDA here in the United States and by equivalent bodies elsewhere in the world. Regulations vary by region, but in general will forbid outright false claims. That's why brands usually can't say a product reduces fine lines and wrinkles without them including at least *some* ingredient that has been shown by research to reduce fine lines and wrinkles.

The problem with this is that these regulations don't attempt to police whether the actual product can produce the results it claims. It just needs to contain ingredients that *can* produce those results, even when those results were achieved under completely different conditions and with the ingredient delivered via a completely different formulation than what is being advertised. So, for example, most studies that demonstrate niacinamide's effectiveness at reducing dark spots and hyperpigmentation used it at a concentration of 4–5%. A product could include niacinamide at a fraction of a single percent yet still claim that it reduces dark spots, simply because its included somewhere in the ingredients list.

Similarly, a product can't claim to include an ingredient that it doesn't (seems obvious). But that doesn't mean it *has* to include the ingredient in any significant amount. Not even if it's the ingredient that the product is named after. Brands are perfectly free to sell "retinol creams" that contain the barest touch of retinol, far less than what is generally required to produce visible changes to skin's texture and appearance. They're also perfectly free to tout the wonders of any particular ingredient, even if the product uses that ingredient in amounts so small they're best expressed in parts per billion.

These are examples of "claims ingredients": ingredients incorporated into a formulation simply to be able to make a claim, instead of included in quantities actually known to affect skin's structure, function, or appearance.

If you remember our discussion about the order in which ingredients are typically arranged on a product label, you'll be unsurprised to find many claims ingredients buried near the bottom of a product's ingredient list. That's not a hard and fast rule, of course, since some ingredients, like retinoids, are effective at very low concentrations, but it is a good rule of thumb to keep in mind when ads attempt to seduce you with talk of their sexy, sexy star ingredients.

The exceptions to these lax advertising regulations are skincare products that fall into the "drug" category rather than the "cosmetics" category. Currently in the US, these include sunscreens, some types of acne medications, and prescription topical medications like tretinoin and higher concentrations of azelaic acid. In those cases, you can feel confident that the product contains sufficient amounts of its active ingredients to reliably produce the effects claimed.

Fear-Based Marketing

Fear-based beauty marketing has dominated the skincare industry for most of the 2010s and has spawned entire new categories of products, most notably the "clean beauty" category.

At its heart, most fear-based beauty marketing operates on the assumption that "chemicals" are dangerous ingredients, usually with long science-y names that many laypeople don't recognize and can't pronounce. It's symptomatic of the larger distrust of science and authority that has led to the creationist, antivax, and climate change denialist movements, but that's beside the point. The point is that it is wildly misleading.

There are intimidating connotations to the word "chemical." To a person without much science education, "chemicals" evokes images of unnatural concoctions dreamed up by heartless scientists in cold, sterile labs—the key term here being "unnatural," because the flip side of the fear of chemicals is the belief that natural substances are inherently safer and better.

First of all, everything is a chemical. It's odd to me to see brands outright claiming their products are "free of chemicals," because every substance that contains matter is a chemical. There are pure chemicals, which consist of molecules that all share the same chemical structure. Water, whose molecules all have two hydrogen atoms and one oxygen atom, is a pure chemical. Plants are made of chemicals, even if they're organically grown according to the purest principles of biodynamic farming. People are also made of chemicals. So are cats, even if they do also contain a little dash of ineffable magic.

Chemicals are neither good nor bad. *Some* chemicals are more beneficial for human health or human skin than others. Other chemicals are less beneficial or more potentially harmful, depending on exposure amounts.

Marketers who tout "chemical free" cosmetics really mean that the products they sell are free of *unnatural* chemicals. Synthetic, manmade substances. The logic is poor here as well. Many manmade or lab-derived substances, like niacinamide, are generally well tolerated and beneficial to skin. Many completely natural substances, on the other hand, are poorly tolerated or of little to no benefit to skin. Poison ivy is an obvious example, but in the realm of natural ingredients you'll find in skincare, some of the best examples are fragrant essential oils used to create a pleasant scent without the addition of artificial fragrance. Fragrant essential oils are known sensitizers for some people,[46] with lemongrass, narcissus, jasmine, and sandalwood oils[47] among the recognized culprits. It's true that the "fragrance" ingredient listed in many products is vague and can be troubling to those who'd like to know exactly what's in their cosmetics. It is not true that naturally derived fragrances pose less risk.

There are some excellent products in the all-natural, organic, or "clean" categories, but the categories themselves exist and profit due to fearmongering and misinformation. If you encounter a product that claims to be free of chemicals, there's no need to dismiss it outright, but neither should you accept any claims of superior safety, gentleness, or effectiveness at face value either. And when you encounter articles in the media about the newly discovered dangers of some common cosmetics ingredient, take a moment to consider the source of the articles' information. Much of the current chemophobia and cosmetics scaremongering originates not from actual scientists and scientific or medical organizations, but from environmental lobbying groups and natural product sellers with a financial interest in pushing the "chemicals bad, nature good" narrative.

THE HEALTHY PURSUIT OF YOUR OWN BEAUTY

Your standards for your own appearance are your own business. I'm not here to unpack or untangle that. It's above my pay grade, and it may not be necessary.

Where you may want to seek professional guidance is if your standards for your personal appearance deviate drastically from what you are physically capable of achieving. If you're short, like me, but are convinced you cannot be beautiful and will not be happy unless you find a way to become tall, that's a problem. If your natural skin tone is deeper but you only see the beauty in porcelain-pale foundation shades, that's something to examine and to work on, perhaps with the help of a qualified therapist.

What we all can work on is recognizing that beauty in the real world, outside of corporate media depictions, comes in all shapes, all colors, all sizes, and all ethnicities. There is no black-and-white cutoff. There is no rule that only those who check off enough boxes on the rubric of conventional beauty will find happiness and fulfillment in life. A healthy pursuit of beauty, one that comes from a place of self-love rather than fear or comparison to others, requires you to pursue the version of beauty that is appropriate and attainable to *you*. The great thing is that the more you recognize this and work towards it, the more you'll see the beauty you already possess.

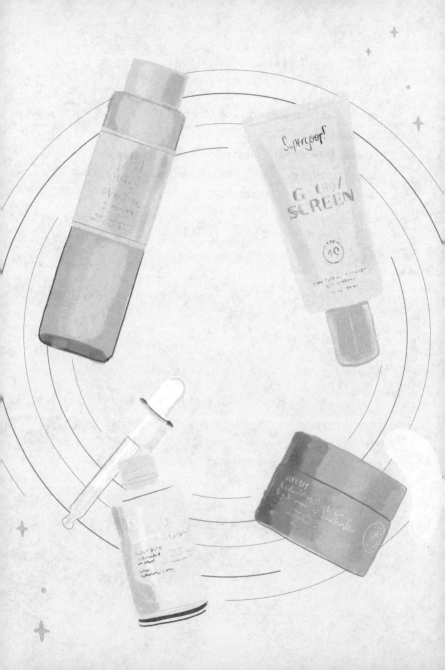

WHERE TO GO FROM HERE

We've reached the end of this book, and I hope I've given you a solid foundation to find your best skincare routine, your best skin, and improved mental health along the way. Before I let you go, though, I want to make sure we're on the same page about some of the most fundamental truths about anyone's skincare journey.

One of the many reasons I've chosen not to mention or recommend specific products in this book is because everyone's skin is different. This doesn't mean that a product that worked for someone else but doesn't work for you is a scam or the other person is a liar; it means that the product that worked for them does not work for you. Just as people have different allergies, food intolerances, and reactions to medications, so too does people's skin respond differently to ingredients.

A glance at even the strongest studies done on the most well established actives shows that nothing has a hundred percent success rate. Nor does any ingredient have a zero percent risk of irritation or breakouts. The best way to learn what your skin likes and what it doesn't like is to pay close attention to how it responds to different products, then figuring out over time which ingredients your best and worst products have in common. As you do so, you'll also be better able to identify the skincare content creators and product reviewers whose skin is most similar to yours. Their recommendations will typically work out better for you than the recommendations of creators with skin that's vastly dissimilar to yours.

Of course, learning these things about your skin takes time, patience, and consistency. Don't let yourself get sucked in to promises of instant or rapid results. Typically, products that promise immediate improvement to skin either achieve it via the use of ingredients that simply mask the skin concerns you're trying to address, or simply won't deliver those results at all. Give every new product an ample amount of time to work on your skin. You will know right away if a cleanser cleanses and a moisturizer moisturizers, but it will likely take weeks to months to see the real effects of most actives or secondary actives. That's a feature, not a bug. As with any other self-improvement regimen, real change takes time and work.

In the meantime, practice being at peace with your own pace of improvement. It's often said that comparison is the thief of joy. This is especially true in beauty, where we're often manipulated into comparing ourselves negatively to others. You are your own standard. How you compare to your next door neighbor, your high school rival, or your favorite film and television actress is irrelevant and ultimately more damaging than inspiring.

Keep the focus on yourself and your own progress. Take progress photos once every couple of weeks if you can, and do them in the same location, at the same angle, and with the same lighting whenever possible. Incremental progress is hard for us to recognize, as I've mentioned before. Having concrete documentation of how far you've come works wonders to remind you that you are on the track (and can help you recognize when you've gone off the rails).

And know that when you approach your skincare and your self-care from a place of love for yourself, you are doing more for yourself than just alleviating dry, uncomfortable skin, clearing up some pimples, or fading a few dark marks here and smoothing out a few fine lines there. What you're doing is demonstrating to yourself that you have value and you deserve care, no matter what your circumstances. You're prioritizing yourself and treating yourself as a person of worth. In the end, that's the best thing you can do for yourself, because it's true.

Take good care of yourself, from your skin inwards!

ACKNOWLEDGEMENTS

People don't develop in a vacuum, and neither do books. Behind my name on the cover is an entire army of friends and colleagues whose support and advice have kept me going and made me better. I'm grateful to them all.

Tracy Robey of *Fanserviced-B*, Chel Cortes of *Holy Snails*, and Cat of *Snow White and the Pear*—all of them also my partners in podcasting crime at *The Snailcast*—were my first, and remain my closest, blogger friends. We've cheered each other on, helped each other up, and served as each other's first readers for so long that I can't imagine being without them.

Kerry Thompson of *Skin and Tonics*, Coco Park of *The Beauty Wolf*, and Sheryll Donerson of *The Wanderlust Project* were the K-beauty bloggers who inspired me the most when I started my blog. I'm fortunate to count them as friends still, and fortunate for the early lucky break I got when Kerry and Coco asked me to contribute my skincare routine to their K-beauty book, *Korean Beauty Secrets: A Practical Guide to Cutting-Edge Skincare and Makeup*.

My fellow crazed cat ladies Angela and Renee from *Beauty and the Cat*, along with Megan and Nicole in our cat lady group chat, help keep me sane and supplied with cat pictures and turtle jokes, no matter how stressed I feel. The annual Christmas shopping pilgrimages to the LA Asian beauty stores with Angela and Renee also provide me with a wealth of material for my blog.

Cheryl Wischhover published my essay on depression and Korean beauty, and Anna Park has published many of my ramblings since; they're some of the best editors and human beings I know.

Actual chemistry PhD Michelle Wong and actual cosmetic chemist Stephen Alain Ko have the patience of saints. I don't have much of a STEM background myself, and they've helped me understand so many concepts that would otherwise have flown right over my heads. They're also genuinely hilarious people. Stephen, my chives would be nothing without your criticism. They know you mean well.

Renee Chow, also known as Gothamista, contributed the foreword for this book and so much happiness to my life. She understands me, and our conversations about skincare, social media, and carbs always leave me feeling like things make sense and I'm not crazy (or alone).

I've had the pleasure of getting to know the teams behind many wonderful beauty brands both large and small over the years. Sulwhasoo, DECIEM, and COSRX hold a special place in my life: my skincare routine is never without their products, and their friendship and support affirms my philosophy that blogging doesn't need to be adversarial. Opportunities arise where interests align, and mine often align with those of these brands.

Finally, my blog would never have gotten off the ground without the support of the Reddit skincare communities between about 2013 to 2016. The encouragement of members over at r/AsianBeauty and r/SkincareAddiction inspired me to keep going; the criticism I sometimes received helped me grow and learn.

ABOUT THE AUTHOR

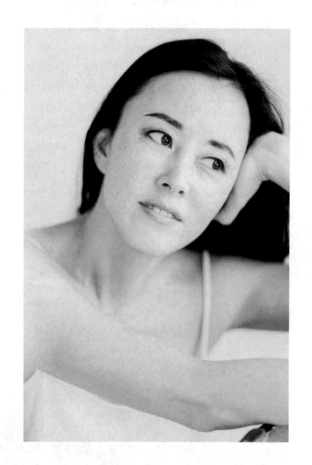

After enlightening but aimless stints in food service, retail, education, and tech journalism, Jude found her calling in skincare—specifically, writing about skincare to share her passion for sunscreen and loathing for overpriced AHAs with the world.

She is known for tying skincare to self-care since the publication of her essay "How My Elaborate Korean Skincare Routine Helps Me Fight Depression" on Fashionista.com in 2015. Since then, she's published steadily, both as a freelance beauty writer and on her blog, Fifty Shades of Snail. Jude has also worked in beauty marketing and consulting for both Korean and American brands.

She has been featured in New York Magazine's The Cut, hailed as "the reigning queen of skincare" by New York Magazine's The Strategist, and included in W's list of "Korean beauty experts you should follow on Instagram." She remains active in online beauty communities, with a large network of like-minded followers and fellow content creators.

ENDNOTES

1 Peter M. Elias, "Stratum Corneum Defensive Functions: An Integrated View," Journal of Investigative Dermatology 125, no 2 (April 2016): 183-200, https://doi.org/10.1111/j.0022-202X.2005.23668.x.

2 K.P. Ananthapadmanabhan, S. Mukherjee, P. Chandar, "Stratum corneum fatty acids: their critical role in preserving barrier integrity during cleansing," International Journal of Cosmetic Science 35, no. 4 (August 2013): 337-345, https://doi.org/10.1111/ics.12042.

3 Michelle Wong, "How to Use Comedogenicity Ratings (With Video)," last modified February 21, 2019, https://labmuffin.com/fact-check-how-to-use-comedogenicity-ratings/

4 K.P. Ananthapadmanabhan, David J. Moore, Kumar Subramanyan, Manoj Misra, "Cleansing without compromise: The impact of cleansers on the skin barrier and the technology of mild cleansing," Dermatologic Therapy 17, no. 1 (February 2004): 16–25, https://doi.org/10.1111/j.1396-0296.2004.04S1002.x.

5 Zoe Diana Draelos MD, "The Science behind skin care: Cleansers," Journal of Cosmetic Dermatology 17, no. 1 (February 2018): 8-14, https://doi.org/10.1111/jocd.12469.

6 "Ultraviolet radiation," World Health Organization, accessed June 17, 2020, https://www.who.int/gho/phe/ultraviolet_radiation/en/.

7 M. A. Farage, K. W. Miller, P. Elsner, H. I. Maibach, "Intrinsic and extrinsic factors in skin ageing: a review," International Journal of Cosmetic Science 30, no. 2 (April 2008): 87-96, https://doi.org/10.1111/j.1468-2494.2007.00415.x.

8   "Sun Protection," Skin Cancer Foundation, accessed August 19, 2020, https://www.skincancer.org/skin-cancer-prevention/sun-protection/.

9   Steve Taylor and Brian Diffey, "Simple dosage guide for suncreens will help users," BMJ (Clinical research ed.) 324 no. 7352 (2002): 1526. doi:10.1136/bmj.324.7352.1526/a.

10 "What is the difference between UVA and UVB rays?," University of Iowa Hospitals & Clinics, accessed August 21, 2020, https://uihc.org/health-topics/what-difference-between-uva-and-uvb-rays.

11 "Sunscreen: How to Help Protect Your Skin from the Sun," U.S. Food & Drug Administration, accessed June 8, 2020, https://www.fda.gov/drugs/understanding-over-counter-medicines/sunscreen-how-help-protect-your-skin-sun.

12 M. Schlumpf, B. Cotton, M. Conscience, V. Haller et al, "In vitro and in vivo estrogenicity of UV Screens," Environmental Health Perspectives, March 2001, https://doi.org/10.1289/ehp.01109239.

13 Henry W. Lim MD, Maria-Ivonne Arellano-Mendoza MD, Fernando Stengel MD, "Current challenges in photoprotection," Journal of the American Academy of Dermatology 76, no. 3 (March 2017):91-99, https://doi.org/10.1016/j.jaad.2016.09.040.

14 Yuki Yamamoto, Koji Uede, Nozomi Yonei, Akiko Kishioka et al., "Effects of alpha-hydroxy acids on the human skin of Japanese subjects: The rationale for chemical peeling," The Journal of Dermatology 33, no. 1 (January 2006): 16-22, https://doi.org/10.1111/j.1346-8138.2006.00003.x.

15 Ryu-Ichiro Hata and Haruki Senoo, "L-ascorbic acid 2-phosphate stimulates collagen accumulation, cell proliferation, and formation of a three-dimensional tissuelike substance by skin fibroblasts," Journal of Cellular Physiology 138, no. 1 (January 1989): 8–16, https://doi.org/10.1002/jcp.1041380103.

16 Steven S. Traikovich, DO, "Use of Topical Ascorbic Acid and Its Effects on Photodamaged Skin Topography," Arch Otolaryngol Head Neck Surg. 125, no. 10 (October 1999): 1091–1098, doi:10.1001/archotol.125.10.1091.

17 K. Graupe, W. J. Cunliffe, H. P. Gollnick, and R. P. Zaumseil, "Efficacy and safety of topical azelaic acid (20 percent cream): an overview of results from European clinical trials and experimental reports," Cutis 57, no. 1 (December 1995): 20–35, https://europepmc.org/article/med/8654128.8

18 R. M. Halder and G. M. Richards, "Topical Agents Used in the Management of Hyperpigmentation," Skin Therapy Letter 9, no. 6 (July 2004), http://www.skintherapyletter.com/hyperpigmentation/topical-agents/.

19 Ella L. Toombs, MD, "Cosmetics in the Treatment of Acne Vulgaris," Dermatologic Clinics 23, no. 3 (July 2005): 575–581, https://doi.org/10.1016/j.det.2005.04.001.

20 Siddharth Mukherjee, Abhijit Date, Vandana Patravale, Hans Christian Korting et al., "Retinoids in the treatment of skin aging: an overview of clinical efficacy and safety," Clin Interv Aging 1, no. 4 (December 2006): 327-348, https://dx.doi.org/10.2147%2Fciia.2006.1.4.327.

21 Loren Pickart, Jessica Michelle Vasquez-Soltero, and Anna Margolina, "GHK Peptide as a Natural Modulator of Multiple Cellular Pathways in Skin Regeneration," BioMed Research International 2015 (2015), https://doi.org/10.1155/2015/648108.

22 "Tripeptide-1," INCI Decoder, accessed October 28, 2020, https://incidecoder.com/ingredients/tripeptide-1.1

23 Loren Pickart, Jessica Michelle Vasquez-Soltero, and Anna Margolina, "GHK-Cu may Prevent Oxidative Stress in Skin by Regulating Copper and Modifying Expression of Numerous Antioxidant Genes," Cosmetics 2, no. 3 (2015): 236-247, https://doi.org/10.3390/cosmetics2030236.

24 Donald L. Bissett, John E. Oblong, and Cynthia A. Berge, "Niacinamide: A B Vitamin that Improves Aging Facial Skin Appearance," Dermatologic Surgery 31, no. 1 (July 2005): 860–866, https://doi.org/10.1111/j.1524-4725.2005.31732.

25 W. Gehring, "Nicotinic acid/niacinamide and the skin," Journal of Cosmetic Dermatology 3, no. 2 (April 2004): 88-93, https://doi.org/10.1111/j.1473-2130.2004.00115.x.

26 A.B. Kimball J.R. Kaczvinsky J. Li L.R. Robinson P.J. Matts et al., "Reduction in the appearance of facial hyperpigmentation after use of moisturizers with a combination of topical niacinamide and N-acetyl glucosamine: results of a randomized, double-blind, vehicle-controlled trial," British Journal of Dermatology 162, no. 2 (February 2010): 435–441, https://doi.org/10.1111/j.1365-2133.2009.09477.x.

27 Maria Valeria Robles Velasco, Vivian Zague, Michelli Dario, and Deborah O. Nishikawa, "Characterization and Short-Term clinical study of clay facial mask," Revista de Ciencias Farmaceuticas Basica e Aplicada 37, no. 1 (January 2016), https://www.researchgate.net/publication/318508286_Characterization_and_Short-Term_clinical_study_of_clay_facial_mask.

28 Grace Tan, Peng Xu, Louise B. Lawson, Jibao He et al., "Hydration Effects on Skin Microstructure as Probed by High-Resolution Cryo-Scanning Electron Microscopy and Mechanistic Implications to Enhanced Transcutaneous Delivery of Biomacromolecules," J Pharm Sci 99, no. 2 (February 2010): 730–740, https://dx.doi.org/10.1002%2Fjps.21863./

29 Wiesława Bylka, Paulina Znajdek-Awiżeń, Elżbieta Studzińska-Sroka, and Małgorzata Brzezińska, "Centella asiatica in cosmetology," Postepy Dermatol Alergol 30, no. 1 (February 2013): 46–49, https://dx.doi.org/10.5114%2Fpdia.2013.33378.

30 Andrew B. Jull, Nicky Cullum, Jo C. Dumville, Maggie J. Westby et al., "Honey as a topical treatment for wounds," Cochrane Systematic Reviews 2015, no. 3 (March 2015): 1465–1458, https://doi.org//10.1002/14651858.CD005083.pub4

31 Tatsuya Ogawa, Yosuke Ishitsuka, Yoshiyuki Nakamura, Naoko Okiyama et al., "Honey and Chamomile Activate Keratinocyte Antioxidative Responses via the KEAP1/NRF2 System," Clin Cosmet Investig Dermatol 2020, no. 13 (September 2020): 657–660, https://dx.doi.org/10.2147%2FCCID.S270602.

32 M. Saeedi, K. Morteza-Semnani, and M. R. Ghoreishi, "The treatment of atopic dermatitis with licorice gel," Journal of Dermatological Treatment 14, no. 3 (July 2009): 153–157, https://doi.org/10.1080/09546630310014369.

33 Giulia Pastorino, Laura Cornara, Sónia Soares, Francisca Rodrigues et al., "Liquorice (Glycyrrhiza glabra): A phytochemical and pharmacological review," Phytotherapy Research 32, no. 12 (December 2018): 2323–2339, https://doi.org/10.1002/ptr.6178.

34 Young-Won Chin, Hyun-Ah Jung, Yue Liu, Bao-Ning Su et al., "Anti-oxidant Constituents of the Roots and Stolons of Licorice (Glycyrrhiza glabra)," J. Agric. Food Chem, 55, no 12 (May 2007): 4691–4697, https://doi.org/10.1021/jf0703553.

35 Kyu Choon Song, Tong-Shin Chang, Hyejin Lee, Jinhee Kim et al., "Processed Panax ginseng, Sun Ginseng Increases Type I Collagen by Regulating MMP-1 and TIMP-1 Expression in Human Dermal Fibroblasts," *Journal of Ginseng Research* 36, no. 1 (2012): 61-67, http://dx.doi.org/10.5142/jgr.2012.36.1.61.

36 Wenyuan Zhu and Jie Gao, "The Use of Botanical Extracts as Topical Skin-Lightening Agents for the Improvement of Skin Pigmentation Disorders," *Journal of Investigative Dermatology Symposium Proceedings* 2008, no. 13 (2008): 20-24, http://dx.doi.org/10.1038/jidsymp.2008.8.

37 Chang-Eui Hong and Su-Yun Lyu, "Anti-inflammatory and Anti-oxidative Effects of Korean Red Ginseng Extract in Human Keratinocytes," Immune Netw. 11, no. 1 (February 2011): 42-49, https://doi.org/10.4110/in.2011.11.1.42.

38 Bruno Bonnemain, "Helix and Drugs: Snails for Western Health Care From Antiquity to the Present," Evid Based Complement Alternat Med 2, no. 1 (March 2005): 25-28, https://dx.doi.org/10.1093%2Fecam%2Fneh057.

39 Agnes Sri Harti, S. Dwi Sulisetyawati, Atiek Murharyati, and Meri Oktariani, "The Effectiveness of Snail Slime and Chitosan in Wound Healing," International Journal of Pharma Medicine and Biological Sciences 5, no. 1 (January 2016): 76-80, http://www.ijpmbs.com/papers/13-E0007.pdf.

40 Sabrina Guillen Fabi, Joel L. Cohen, Jennifer D. Peterson, Monika G. Kiripolsky et al., "The Effects of Filtrate of the Secretion of the Cryptomphalus Aspersa on Photoaged Skin," J Drugs Dermatol. 12, no. 4 (April 2013): 453-457, https://pubmed.ncbi.nlm.nih.gov/23652894/.

41 Olamide Sanusi, "8 Reasons You Should Try Snail Slime On Your Skin," The Guardian, September 23, 2019, https://guardian.ng/life/8-reasons-you-should-try-snail-slime-on-your-skin/.

42 L. Guilloux D.-A. Vuitton M. Delbourg A. Lagier et al., "Cross-reactivity between terrestrial snails (Helix species) and house-dust mite (Dermatophagoides pteronyssinus). II. In vitro study," Allergy 53, no. 2 (February 1998): 151–158, https://doi.org/10.1111/j.1398-9995.1998.tb03863.x.x

43 Valentina Jesumani, Hong Du, Muhammad Aslam, Pengbing Pei et al., "Potential Use of Seaweed Bioactive Compounds in Skincare—A Review," Mar Drugs 17, no. 2 (December 2019): 688, https://dx.doi.org/10.3390%2Fmd17120688./

44 Michelle Wong, https://www.instagram.com/reel/CGw_sqXnuAB/

45 Christopher Iriarte, Olabola Awosika, Monica Rengifo-Pardo, and Alison Ehrlich, "Review of applications of microneedling in dermatology," Clin. Cosmet. Investig. Dermatol. 2017, no. 10 (August 2017): 289-298, https://dx.doi.org/10.2147%2FCCID.S142450.

46 Narelle Bleasel, Bruce Tate, and Marius Rademaker, "Allergic contact dermatitis following exposure to essential oils," Australasian Journal of Dermatology 43, no. 3 (August 2002): 211–213, https://doi.org/10.1046/j.1440-0960.2002.00598.x.

47 P. J. Frosch, J. D. Johansen, T. Menné, C. Pirker et al., "Further important sensitizers in patients sensitive to fragrances," Contact Dermatitis 47, no. 5 (November 2002): 279–287, https://doi.org/10.1034/j.1600-0536.2002.4704171.x.

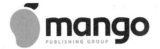

Mango Publishing, established in 2014, publishes an eclectic list of books by diverse authors—both new and established voices—on topics ranging from business, personal growth, women's empowerment, LGBTQ studies, health, and spirituality to history, popular culture, time management, decluttering, lifestyle, mental wellness, aging, and sustainable living. We were named 2019 and 2020's #1 fastest growing independent publisher by Publishers Weekly. Our success is driven by our main goal, which is to publish high quality books that will entertain readers as well as make a positive difference in their lives.

Our readers are our most important resource; we value your input, suggestions, and ideas. We'd love to hear from you—after all, we are publishing books for you!

Please stay in touch with us and follow us at:

Facebook: Mango Publishing

Twitter: @MangoPublishing

Instagram: @MangoPublishing

LinkedIn: Mango Publishing

Pinterest: Mango Publishing

Newsletter: mangopublishinggroup.com/newsletter

Join us on Mango's journey to reinvent publishing, one book at a time.